Pregnancy and Oral Health

The critical connection between your mouth and your baby

Sheila Wolf, RDH

"Mama Gums"

R

Radcliffe Publishing

San Diego, California

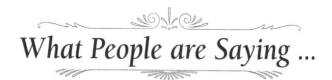

What People are Saying ...

"Sheila Wolf, a hygienist with over 32 years of experience in the practice of preventive dentistry, has written a book filled with clear, practical information that can have immediate as well as long-term benefits on the dental health of all readers, especially that of mothers-to-be. Ms. Wolf's book distills findings from many years of clinical and laboratory research into an easily understood handbook for the prevention and control of the bacterial infections that cause tooth-decay, gingivitis, and periodontitis. With careful professional supervision, the self-care measures she describes should provide excellent dental health for a lifetime. Her book is a vital contribution to our nation's oral health."

Dr. Paul H. Keyes, D.D.S., M.S., F.A.C.D., esteemed former senior researcher in the Institute for Dental Research at the National Institutes of Health.

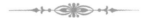

"The message of this book is eye opening. Its potentially life-altering information is at the very least as important to share as the experiences we women have always shared with our expectant daughters, acquaintances, and friends. This book is a must read for every woman. Moreover, it should be in the office of every obstetrician-gynecologist."

Elinor Ruth Smith, Educational Consultant, Teacher Educator

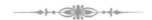

"Mama Gums' book contains sound practical advice backed by scientific evidence to help preserve oral health in harmony with nature."

Dr. Russell C. Tontz, Dentist

"Pre-Term Low Birth Weight Babies cost the people of the United States untold billions of dollars every year, and it is over 7 times more prevalent in those women with periodontal infection. Mama-Gums' book will show you how to prevent and/or treat this infection before it causes damage. I can enthusiastically recommend this book to anyone interested in healthier babies!"

Dr. Thomas Baldwin, DDS, MAGD, F/AIAOMT, BS in Psychology, Masters in Holistic Nutrition, Clayton College of Natural Health, in process.

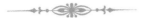

"I had no idea that I'd worry so much, about seemingly everything, during my pregnancy, but I am happy to say that I found Mama Gums' book early on, so I haven't had to add pregnancy gingivitis and its related complications to the list. Moreover, I have learned so much from the book that I feel confident that I will be able to maintain a healthy mouth for life."

Jayne Amani, Attorney, mother-to-be

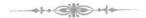

"This is a must-read for all pregnant women. Sheila Wolf has brought together, in one easy-to-read book, the advice of experts in many health fields. If you want a healthy baby, this is the book to read!"

Bill Landers, President, Oratec Corporation

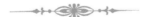

"This book was interesting and informative. I wish it had been written during my pregnancy. I could have avoided the many problems I had with my teeth and gums and I would have saved myself a bunch of money."

Nina Weber, former patient

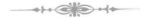

"Excellent. Very informative and entertaining. What a great balance. Readers will thoroughly enjoy it."

Martha Fischer, Teacher

Radcliffe Publishing
Post Office Box 151708
San Diego, CA 92175-1708

First Edition 2004
Library of Congress Catalog Number: 2003092381
International Standard Book Number: 0-9740528-0-9

Library of Congress Cataloging in Publication Data

Wolf, Sheila.
Pregnancy and oral health : the critical connection between your mouth and your baby / Sheila Wolf, "Mama Gums". -- 1st ed.
p. cm.
Includes bibliographical references and index.
LCCN 2003092381
ISGN 0-9740528-0-9

1. Gums--Diseases--Popular works. 2. Pregnancy--Complications--Popular works. I. Title.

RK401.W65 2004   617.6'32'00852
                   QB103-200834

The cover photograph and the photographs within are the copyrighted work of Heather Van Gaale, and are used with her permission. Further examples of Heather's beautiful, intimate, non-traditional portraits can been seen at her web site at: www.blinkphoto.com.

Illustrations and graphic designs by Bonnie Thompson
www.findcreative.com/web/bonthompson/index.html

Book layout and design by: Jean Savage, JGS Designs
                           Eva Urick, Urick Design: www.urickdesign.com

Clipart images from Dover. All rights reserved.

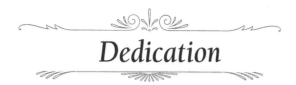

Dedication

This book is dedicated to all of my wonderful clients, patients, and friends who have taught me so much through the years, not only about dentistry, but also about love and communication

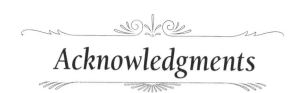

Acknowledgments

Bravo to those brave and innovative thinkers, researchers, scholars, and educators who have looked outside the box for new ways of treating gum disease. They include: first and foremost, Dr. Paul H. Keyes, "an inquisitive maverick" who has generously given of his time to read this book and offer suggestions, and Dr. Dan Watt, a respected teacher and mentor, both founders of the International Dental Health Foundation.

Some early pioneers: Dr. Paul Cummings, Dr. Thomas Hartzell, Dr. Walter Loesche, Dr. Thomas Rams, Dr. Jorgen Slots, Dr. Sigmund Socransky, Dr. Max Listgarten, Dr. Lawrence Page, Dr. Jason Tanzer, Dr. Jasim Albander, Dr. Daniel Fine, Dr. Ernest Newbrun, Dr. Ulf Wikesjo, Dr. Richard Ellen, Dr. R. Leslie Arnett, Dr. I. Stephen Brown, Dr. Roger J. Forman, Dr. Thomas McCawley, Dr. Irving Romanow, Dr. Norman Trieger, Dr. James Giordano, Dr. Robert Genco, Dr. Vincent M. Cali, Dr. Jerome Hill, Dr. Larry Burnett, Dr. Jim Knott, Dr. Irv Lubis and Dr. David Kennedy.

Friends and mentors who read the book and gave me wonderful feedback and advice: Dr. Robert White, Dr. Russell C. Tontz, Dr. Tom Baldwin, and Dr. Barry Solomon. I also recognize all the past and present members of the International Dental Health Foundation, Claire Friedlander, and all those courageous practitioners and researchers who dared to be different.

Also to be acknowledged are the scientists, researchers, and professionals whose work includes uncovering the evidence in the link between gum infections and adverse pregnancy outcomes. Amongst them are: Dr. Steven Offenbacher, Dr. Jim Beck, Dr. Marjorie Jeffcoat, and Dr. Nestor Lopez.

To my editor, Rusty Fischer, thank you for your participation in the editing and in the promotion of this book. I appreciate your wonderful sense of humor and your good-natured, cheerful reactions to whatever wild ideas I may have. You have been my "rock."

Thank you, Heather Van Gaale, for contributing your stunning and unique maternity photographs showcased in this book.

I thank all the people who were willing to contribute their time, their words of wisdom, and their personal comments to add to the value of this book.

Thank you Bill Landers from Oratec for contributing your wisdom, your incredible knowledge, your editing, and your friendship. I also appreciate your enthusiasm when asked to add your "two cents."

I thank Dr. Harold Horton, now retired and living in Florida, and Dr. David Millen, still practicing periodontics in New Haven, Connecticut, for their superb training in the basics of dental hygiene and for a nearly 20-year relationship. I also thank Dr. Sheldon Natkin for his support in my early years as a hygienist.

Dr. Peter K. Hellwig, thank you for giving me the permission I needed to freely express my creativity in my dentistry as I do so easily in other areas of my life. You are very special, and I thank you for making the last third of my career as a hygienist the most gratifying of all.

I am grateful to my remarkable mother, Nora Wolf, who lives her life with courage and enthusiasm. Unstopped by circumstances, she has managed to pursue multiple careers, start businesses, and travel the world. Whew! Thanks, Mom, for being such a role model for me. A great big hug!

I thank my precious son, Alan Ranciato, who has always been so much wiser than his chronological years, for freely bestowing on me his incredible good judgment, support, feedback, and encouragement. Honey, you are so special.

I remember with appreciation, my loving father, Albert Wolf, who listened to my dreams and aspirations and strongly encouraged me to express my creativity, especially in the kitchen.

I appreciate my maternal grandmother, Tania Toplitsky, a unique and colorful musician, raconteur, entertainer and writer who was important in shaping who I am.

I thank my beloved SMEF group, Elinor Ruth Smith, Marty Saul, and Flewid Kahn for their coaching, love, and friendship. I thank Jayne Amani, who gave me feedback from a pregnant mom's perspective.

Another special thanks goes to Bonnie Marie Thompson for her wonderful illustrations and Jean Savage and Eva Urick for the layout and design of the book.

There are many extraordinary people and organizations that have contributed to my growth and development and offered validation, support, clarity, and mentorship along my life path and through this project: Werner Erhard, Landmark Education Corporation, Income Builders International (IBI), Avrom King, the teachers of The Optimum Health Institute, and my potpourri of spiritual advisors through the years. Other supportive friends include: Sabrina Mizrahi, Hans Zandee, Sharry Mickels, Debbie Webb, Judy Salsbery, Darlene Evans, Susan Stout and Mark Rickett, Amy Anding McClure, Maggie Johnson from Nexadental, John Sullivan from WL Gore, Sarah Ann Telles, Ellis Whitcomb, Nancy Worchester, Kikuno Miller, Hildy Kahn, Eric Gibson, Mim Goloboff, Allen Lowrimore, David Cameron Kirsch, Chris Joiner, Tim Darrell Hillman, Jacob Princeton Regal, Dr. Michael Ryce, Amy Munson, Louis and Sheila Vazquez, Jeff and Rebecca Kurtz, Mike McCarthy, Jessica Clark, Nancee Hanson, Sandie and Marc Taylor, Dr. Ann Louise Gittleman, Billie Gray, Esq., Dr. Marvin A. Steinberg, and anyone else I forgot to mention … forgive me.

And to my partner, Ian Radcliffe. Thank you for your belief in me and for your support in the development of this book. I appreciate so many things about you, not the least being your amazing talent for words, your invaluable assistance with the organization, research, proofreading, and editing, as well as your constant encouragement and moral support throughout this project.

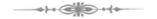

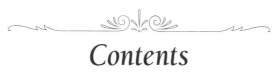

Contents

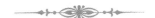

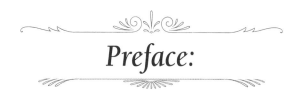

Preface:

Why I Wrote This Book

I have been treating gum diseases now for more than thirty years. Along with a growing number of dental professionals, I have seen evidence of the vital connection between the health of the mouth and the health of the body as a whole. In May of 2000, *Oral Health in America: A Report of the Surgeon General* defined this connection, linking the "silent epidemic" of gum disease with increased risk of serious diseases such as heart attack, stroke, diabetes, ulcers, respiratory problems, and adverse pregnancy outcomes like premature birth and low birth weight babies. In the last chapter of the report, *A Call to Action,* the Surgeon General makes a plea to all health professionals and educators to "enhance the public's understanding of oral health and the relationship of the mouth to the rest of the body."

My life's work has been about empowering people to take control of their whole body wellness by achieving and maintaining excellent oral health. It seemed a natural next step to reach out past the limited numbers who sit in my dental chair and make this information available to everyone.

In the course of researching and writing about a disease that impacts 4 out of 5 Americans, I sent an article on pregnancy and oral health to several women's web sites. I was delighted by their enthusiastic response. They were eager to share this information with their readership because there is almost nothing out there informing women about the critical connection between their oral health and the health of their unborn babies.

Despite the impact of oral health on general health and well being, the mouth is often overlooked or ignored by doctors and left to us dental professionals. In all the years that I have had routine physicals, I have never had a doctor once look in my mouth to perform an oral exam. To peek at my tonsils, yes. But never to check out my gums, my teeth, my tongue, or even to look for oral cancer. In my experience, OB/GYNs, specializing in women and maternity issues, don't generally get involved in concerns of the mouth either. Even in the dental profession, outside of a small group of holistic and naturopathic dentists, I have found few who look beyond the mouth and involve the patient in participating in his or her own wellness.

This brings up important questions. Whose responsibility is it to give advice to a prospective mother about what she can expect in her oral tissues, given the hormonal changes in her body? Who will explain to her the **why** and the **how to** of the special care needed to minimize the bacterial diseases that often develop during pregnancy? How will she know that such infections during this time can influence the health of the baby she carries? I wanted to take on this project to support moms in having the safest pregnancies and the healthiest babies possible.

In the United States alone, more than four million babies are born every year, giving me the opportunity to contribute to countless women, families, and unborn children, and to transform the quality of people's lives. Thanks to all you expectant Moms for providing me this wonderful opportunity to make a difference and share in your joyous occasion.

God bless.

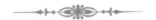

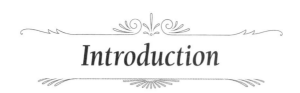

Introduction

We often take our mouths for granted; yet our mouths are the essence of our humanity. Aside from the obvious, breathing, eating, chewing, and swallowing, our mouths are the way we communicate to the world. We smile at each other, speak gentle words of love, convey our feelings for one another, sigh a breath of relief, cry out in joy or in pain, chew, taste, kiss our beloved, express our sexuality, share from our hearts, and communicate our deepest thoughts with facial expressions.

The mouth is often what impacts a stranger on a first impression. A smile invites, a frown deflects. We see youth and vitality in a set of gleaming, lustrous teeth. There is so much that "speaks" to us when a healthy, fresh smelling, kissable mouth gives us a "hello." There is a wealth of information we see in the mouth even before we hear the utterance of words.

In Chinese medicine, the mouth is an important indicator of the health of the body. The mouth is also a portal of entry to the body and an important structure of survival. If the internal coverings of the mouth, the literal "skin" of our cheeks, gums, tongue etc., are broken or compromised in any way, the mouth becomes a conduit through which bacteria, viruses, and other threatening invaders make their way into the inner sanctuary of the body.

It is naïve to assume one can be healthy when something is wrong with the mouth. In *Oral Health in America* the Surgeon General tells us, "Oral health is integral to general health. You cannot be healthy without oral health. Oral health and general health should not be interpreted as separate entities."

Recent studies indicate that as many as four out of five Americans suffer from some form of gum disease. While many have only the early forms such as gingivitis, these relatively mild gum infections often lead to periodontitis, which attacks the tissues and bone that form the very foundation for your teeth.

Periodontal diseases, now known as periodontal *infections*, put your very teeth squarely at risk. Sufficiently advanced, these bacterial infections will cause teeth to become loose, or even to fall out altogether. In fact, 60% of all lost adult teeth are victims, not of tooth decay, but of these insidious gum infections.

Ask anyone who's ever had it happen. Tooth loss definitely impacts your quality of life. For example, I once had a patient who was terrified that if she either sneezed or coughed her dentures would be propelled out of her mouth and go flying across the room! Needless to say, that consciousness affected her every social activity. The ravages of these insidious bacterial infections may adversely affect not just your smile, but also your very self-image and self-worth.

Yet this is arguably not the most important part of the story. The Surgeon General's May 2000 Report was prompted in part by the growing bodies of evidence linking gum disease with a number of life-threatening illnesses including adverse pregnancy outcomes.

- *Periodontal disease is an infection, and all infections are dangerous to pregnant women because they pose a threat to the health of the baby.*

- *Pregnant women with periodontal disease are seven times more likely to have pre-term, low birth weight babies.*

- *Low birth weight has been related to 60% of infant deaths.*

- *There can be up to a three times greater risk of stroke and heart attack for people with severe periodontal disease.*

- *Mouth bacteria have been found to be responsible for fifty-five percent of cases of infectious edema (swelling from bacterial infection).*

By teaching generations of patients the correct techniques, recommending the most effective tools, and expanding oral hygiene to include a campaign of **"antibacterial warfare"** that will rid the body of infection, I have helped many to keep their teeth, improve their health, and avoid costly and invasive surgeries that other professionals recommended, often after calling their condition "hopeless." The work we are going to do together is based on holistic principles and will teach you a simple, economical, ten-minute-a-day program of self-care that will enable you to enjoy good health for both yourself and your baby.

The body has an inherent ability to make itself well. By removing the microorganisms that cause infection, we create an environment where the body can naturally heal itself. We are going to address the underlying causes of the infections, acknowledge that this is a whole body problem (since the body is affected by all its systems), and then remove obstacles to health and recovery. This is an opportunity to take an active role in your own health.

What is available to you is to keep your natural teeth for your lifetime, and to achieve optimum health and wellness for your mouth, your body, and your unborn baby. From there, oral health and well being become available to your children ... and their children as well.

You are now on your way ...

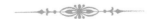

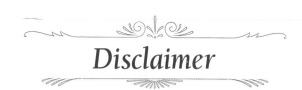

Disclaimer

The information, guidelines, instructions, and opinions that I have presented in this book are based upon the work of our forefathers in microscopy, the May 2000 report of the Surgeon General of the United States, entitled *Oral Health in America,* and the findings of countless other dedicated researchers involved in studies linking gum diseases with many of the systemic illnesses that plague our society today, including those specific to pregnant women. I have also included what I have learned from my experiences of more than thirty years in clinical periodontal care, working with thousands of patients on a more natural, holistic, and non-surgical approach to periodontal therapy.

It is not my intention to diagnose or prescribe. Nor are these writings intended to replace the advice of a qualified dental or medical professional. If you have any questions as to the appropriateness of any of the opinions, suggestions, or information contained in this book, please consult your obstetrician, gynecologist, dentist, periodontist, or other health specialist.

This book is not intended to be a substitute for professional dental advice — only a helping hand down the path to periodontal health.

Are you ready to follow me there?

Good. Let's get started…

Chapter One

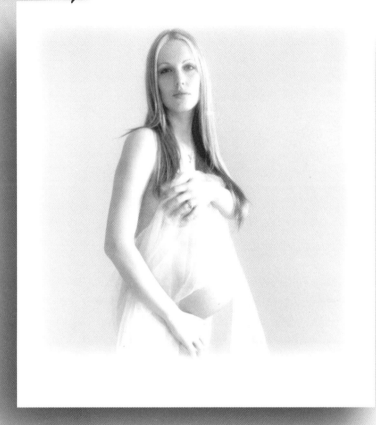

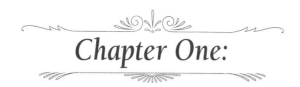

Chapter One:

The "Scope" of the Problem

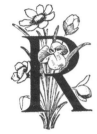ain was falling steadily that crisp September day in 1971, when I first stepped into the hallowed hallways of Fones School of Dental Hygiene. Like so many other young, independent women of my generation, I was about to embark on a career of my own, never expecting it to continue for thirty-two years. During my career, the field of dentistry has seen many changes, the biggest of which has been the recognition of the role that bacteria play in gum disease and tooth decay.

I chuckle when I remember that I began my career before OSHA, (Occupational Safety and Health Administration) when everything in the dental operatory was considered acceptable as long as it was "kitchen clean." No gloves, no masks. No AIDS.

For the first twenty years of my career, I worked in one of the first periodontal practices in New Haven, Connecticut, a prestigious office with very high standards of care. I scraped tartar and polished stains off people's teeth during their maintenance visits, encouraged them to brush and floss, looked for cavities, and talked about gum disease.

Despite our very high standards, it was frustrating to see that we weren't really helping all our patients get healthy. In many, their routine x-rays clearly disclosed bone loss that had progressed to a point at which they were advised to have gum surgery to delay losing their teeth.

At that time, periodontal surgery was the *usual* option we had to prevent loss of teeth from periodontal diseases. After undergoing what now seems to be a radical and unnecessarily invasive mode of treatment, some patients *did* stay healthier for a while after surgery, but too many slipped back into an infected state that often required even *more* surgery.

Many pregnant women developed *pregnancy gingivitis*, a painful condition of the gums exacerbated by the hormones of pregnancy. After a period of time without appropriate attention, this gingivitis commonly evolved into a more serious problem called *periodontitis*, the consequences of which included the loss of teeth and the destruction of bone in the jaw.

There is an old wives' tale that suggests that a woman will lose one tooth for every child. With what we now know about the disease process in the mouth, it doesn't have to be that way. I am now convinced that any woman with an acute oral infection can take control *before* and even *while* she is pregnant, preventing this infection from affecting her mouth for the rest of her life, and also from impacting her pregnancy.

A Bacterial Infection

In 1990, I moved across the continent and began practicing dental hygiene in an innovative California office. There, I encountered a new philosophy based on the work of Dr. Paul H. Keyes, Senior Dental Researcher at the National Institutes of Health, and I learned to use a new and powerful medical device, a *phase contrast microscope*, which I had heard about only superficially.

Phase Contrast Microscope

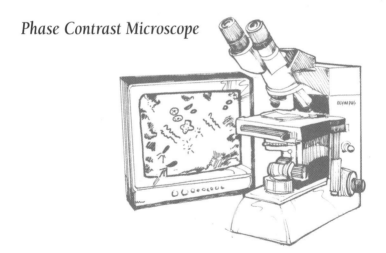

There was a provocative idea circulating that **bacteria** caused gum diseases, not the tartar that I had painstakingly scraped off the teeth all these years. Technically, in a periodontal infection, it is not the bacteria in the plaque that cause the bone loss, but rather the body's reaction to the bacterial toxins, encouraging the immune system to start the process of inflammation. This inflammatory process ultimately results in the loss of the teeth.

The idea that bacteria existed between the teeth wasn't new. As long ago as the late 1600s, a Dutch scientist named Antony Van Leeuwenhoek discovered these squirming, wormlike "animalcules" under one of the first microscopes. However, their connection with gum disease and tooth loss was still rather far off. Who ever could have imagined that there would be more than 500 species of microorganisms discovered in the mouth?

In 1976, Dr. Walter Loesche, then professor of Microbiology and Immunology at the University of Michigan's School of Dentistry, introduced a new concept in the etiology (causation) of periodontal diseases. He asserted that **all plaques are not considered equal**, that **specific** bacteria are responsible for periodontal infections. This is very significant, and his insight revolution-ized the diagnosis and treatment of dento-bacterial disease. It explains why brushing, flossing, and twice a year dental "cleanings", the accepted treatments that are still taught in dental schools around the world, don't work … and why 75% of the population has mouth infections. Rather than just reducing the generalized mass of plaque in the mouth, we must manage the *specific* microor-ganisms to eliminate dental infections. Dr. Loesche developed the BANA test, an easy, practical, five-minute chair side method of testing for these pathogenic bacteria. (See "Specific Plaque Hypothesis" in the Glossary to learn the names of the culprits.)

Using an upgraded, twentieth-century "scope" and a TV monitor to view plaque from under the gingival crevices (the areas under the gums), I can show my patients some of the billions of germs responsible for their gum infections. They are often mesmerized — and certainly disturbed — to see all the activity of the "little world" in their mouths, a miniature society of germ life, all living, feeding, and reproducing under their gum tissues. A few have even said to me that the bacteria seem to be "having a party," and I have been known to answer wryly on such occasions, "Yes, and guess who is the **host**?"

I find that this exciting part of treatment, co-discovering the source of infection, looking at the bacteria (both good and bad) under the microscope, and having patients "own them" and take responsibility for them, is the first step in treating their infections. Each time they come in for treatment, we observe their microscopic "bad guys" and applaud as their numbers and activity diminish, until ultimately they have been eliminated.

Patients are motivated and empowered to take control of their own mouths. They soon have confirmation that their simple, ten-minute-a-day self-care program really works. They may use disclosing tablets or solution, containing a harmless red dye, that reveals how effectively they have been removing the surface bacteria from their teeth and gums. They participate with

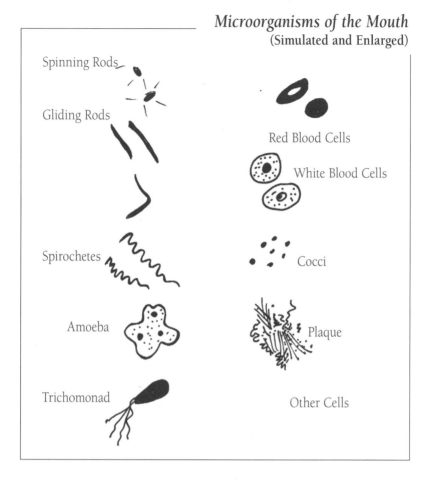

Microorganisms of the Mouth
(Simulated and Enlarged)

Spinning Rods

Gliding Rods

Red Blood Cells

White Blood Cells

Spirochetes

Cocci

Amoeba

Plaque

Trichomonad

Other Cells

pride and enthusiasm as co-therapists, working as a team member, rather than waiting to be "fixed" by us professionals every six months.

I also teach them that those pesky bacteria that cause periodontal infections are contagious, transmissible through kissing and through the exchange of saliva. I invite them to bring in their spouses or partners so that both can be treated.

Again, being pregnant presents its unique oral challenges. Because of the radical hormonal changes of pregnancy, an expectant mothers' gum tissues become more vulnerable to infection. This not only affects her mouth, but also has far-reaching consequences to her whole body health in addition to her pregnancy and her unborn child.

If I have been a good teacher and coach, the expectant mother whom I have educated, trained, and inspired in the **mechanics** and **chemistry** of effective self-care, will properly and enthusiastically disinfect her mouth every day and never have to lose even one tooth through disease. She will take control, and thus increase her chances of having a healthy pregnancy and a healthy baby.

So, reminding myself about that rainy day back in 1971, I'm glad I stuck around for all these years to see and enjoy the progress we have made in dental health. What a privilege to be in this wonderful helping profession and to continue to contribute to the quality of people's lives.

Now, let's start with yours ...

Wow! My Pregnancy Test is Positive!

That is the reaction you might have had upon first learning the good news. You are flooded with excitement at this new discovery, while at the same time experiencing terror at the very thought of it, especially if this is your first time. So many emotions surge through you as you envision and anticipate the next nine months.

So, now that you know for sure, you will naturally be concerned with preparing your body to nurture this new life you are expecting. You will want to consider going to childbirth classes; the support and friendships you will encounter there will be wonderful. You will probably find yourself reading all the books you can lay your hands on to answer the many questions you will undoubtedly have.

You will most likely be selecting a doctor, chatting with your mother, sisters, girlfriends, and neighbors to get their guidance, draw on their wisdom, and find out what you can expect in the coming months. You may even decide to attend La Leche League classes to learn more about breast-feeding. All of these resources, and many more, will facilitate your fascinating journey through this new adventure.

You already know about some of the physical changes you will experience. We all recognize the protruding belly or the posture of a woman close to delivering her baby. Perhaps you are not as familiar with the subtle changes that will take place in your body, however. Many of these changes, such as new freckles or patterns of pigmentation of your skin, and perhaps the loss of sheen in your hair, come from the production of special hormones that prepare your body for the journey ahead.

Hormonal Changes Bring Surprises

On at least three separate occasions, I can remember having the privilege of breaking the news of a young woman's pregnancy from my side of the dentist's chair. I use the word "privilege" with my tongue planted firmly in my cheek, however. After all, the diagnosis was only determined because of the patient's distinctively red, tender, and very swollen gums.

Ouch!

Talk about taking the good news with the bad.

Known as *pregnancy gingivitis*, this unpleasant condition is often assumed to be one of the natural consequences of the hormonal changes found in pregnant women. The hormones involved, estrogen and progesterone, are secreted in progressively greater concentrations throughout most of pregnancy. This flood of hormones results in a variety of effects.

Hormones tell the kidneys to retain water in order to build blood volume to have enough to nourish the placenta. Thus a pregnant woman has 40% more fluid in her body. As a result, this increases the amount of fluid in all the cells in the body, including the gum tissues, which causes them to become puffy and spongy. Between the time of conception and the seventh month of pregnancy, hormones will triple in quantity, and then remain at that heightened level until delivery.

Most mothers-to-be have no idea of the changes that occur in their mouths at this time. Although some doctors, dentists, and hygienists may be aware of these changes, they have rarely received formal education that teaches them how to manage a woman's **oral** health during pregnancy. Consequently, I am going to teach you what is important not only for you as a Mom, but also (according to research studies around the world) what is just as important for your baby.

As Dr. Thomas Rams, professor and chairman of the Department of Periodontology at Temple University School of Dentistry in Philadelphia, points out, "There are hormonal shifts in pregnancy that reduce the gingival tissue resistance to infection, and there is also an increased risk that the hormones circulating will help promote the growth of certain bacteria and plaque, which causes inflammation." Rams also says, "In periodontitis, bacterial plaque infection not only causes inflammation of gingival tissues like gingivitis, but also progressively destroys connective tissue fibers and surrounding bone anchoring teeth to the jaws, resulting in the loss of teeth."

Knowing how to minimize the bacterial biofilms in your mouth, and especially along the gum margins and crevices, is the key factor in preventing pregnancy gingivitis and the escalation of infection that often continues after pregnancy. Ideally, a woman needs to be taught the self-care measures that control the tiny critters that cause periodontitis *before* she gets pregnant. I want to reassure you again, however, that it is never too late. You can reverse pregnancy gingivitis. Dr. Steven Offenbacher, distinguished professor of the UNC School of Dentistry confirms, "Periodontal diseases are both preventable and treatable."

As if she doesn't have enough to contend with, the pregnant woman's tender, swollen gums make it difficult to do an effective job with self-care. When gums become painful and puffy, and bleed during pregnancy, the tendency is to avoid touching them. However, it is imperative that you practice good oral hygiene during pregnancy to avoid both tooth decay and gum infections. Pregnancy, with its three-fold increase in hormones, exacerbates the body's normal response to bacteria, but this need not increase your risk of getting gum disease.

Remember, it is the body's immune response to the *bacterial infections*, not the hormones themselves, that causes the gingivitis. Despite the fact that 50-75% of all pregnant women develop pregnancy gingivitis, *you* do not have to become a statistic. Even if you are already pregnant, I am pleased to tell you that with proper self-care, (using techniques, tools, and medicaments that you may not have learned before reading this book) pregnancy gingivitis can be prevented and controlled.

Although relatively rare, the body's response to inflammation may produce a pregnancy "tumor" (called *pyogenic granuloma*). This "tumor" may develop on the gums in response to the irritating bacteria that collect there. Rest assured, however, that these growths of extra tissue are usually painless, and totally benign. However, if they get large enough, these "pregnancy tumors" can become annoying and should be treated. Meticulous plaque control is the answer to avoiding these growths, and if you do have one, it is comforting to know that they usually subside after childbirth.

Maintaining good oral health is imperative at this significant time in your life. According to the Surgeon General's Report, studies have shown that, "Severe periodontal disease was associated with a seven-fold increase in risk of low birth weight, after controlling for known risk factors such as smoking, race, alcohol use, age, nutrition, and genitourinary tract infection ... suggesting an association between periodontal disease and prematurity."

Other studies from the Report indicate "a link between oral infection and changes in the fetal environment. Toxins or other products generated by the bacteria from periodontal infections may reach the general circulation, cross the placenta, and harm the fetus." The mother's immune system, fighting the infection in her mouth, may actually "interfere with fetal growth and delivery." It is the infection that seems to trigger chemicals called prostaglandins that induce premature delivery.

You may already have a gum infection. You may develop one. You certainly will want to be watchful at this crucial time. If you have any suspicions as to the status of your oral health, take this little test. If you answer, "yes" to even one of these questions, you should be concerned and consider that you probably already have an infection.

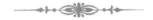

Do I Have a Gum Infection? Take the Test:

1. Are your gums tender, swollen, painful, or itchy?

2. Do your gums ever bleed when you brush your teeth or when you use a toothpick?

3. Are your teeth feeling loose?

4. Have you noticed any spaces developing between your teeth or do they seem to be moving?

5. Are your gums receding (pulling away from your teeth)?

6. Are you troubled with constant bad breath?

7. Have you noticed pus oozing out from your gums when you press on them?

8. Have you noticed any changes in your bite or in the fit of your partial denture?

Brushing, flossing, and irrigating daily (all done gently but deliberately) are important in preventing gingivitis during pregnancy and anytime in your life. If your gums are tender and brushing is painful, try ice, or several helpful over-the-counter products that will sooth painful gums. (Be sure to ask your medical doctor if he or she has objections to any of these products.) These include:

+ Therasol®
+ Orajel® Mouth-Aid
+ Gly-oxide®
+ Peroxyl® Mouth Rinse
+ Amosan® Oral Rinse
+ Anbesol® Liquid
+ Warm salt water

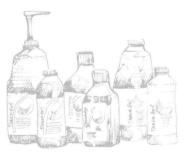

Therasol®

Notes

Chapter Two

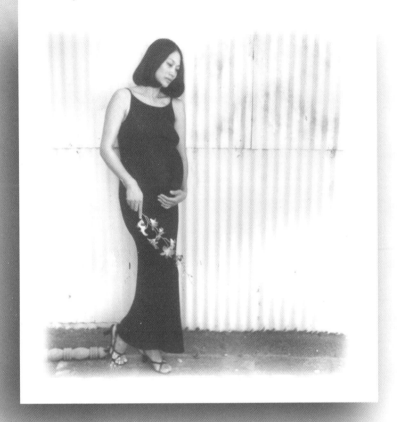

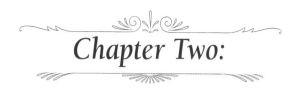

Chapter Two:

Brushing Up

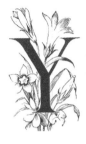ou are about to transform the relationship you have probably had your entire life to cleaning your teeth. If you are like me, when you think of cleaning, you probably think of dirt. I clean the dirt off my car. Your mouth is not dirty like your car, your windows, or your kitchen floor. It doesn't have dust and grime. Rather, your mouth contains a tiny world of bacteria, a very complex society of microorganisms, not unlike a little city in the ways its residents work together and support each other's activities.

There are over 500 different kinds of tiny and varied species of germ life so small they can only be viewed with a microscope or identified from bacterial cultures in a laboratory. This collection of microbes is composed of billions of teeny-tiny microscopic "bugs," some good, some bad.

Left to themselves and undisturbed, the bad bugs can develop into pathogenic (disease-causing) plaques or *biofilms* that live on your teeth, their roots, and the areas around them, under your gums. If not controlled, specific bugs may cause the infections that break down your teeth and the supporting structures that hold your teeth in your jaws.

Today, we know that tooth decay, gum diseases, abscesses, pus, and bone loss are all caused by bacterial infections. Brushing and flossing, the traditional means of *mechanically* cleaning your teeth, are just not enough. If they were enough, three quarters of the population of the United States would not have gum diseases and the risks of systemic illnesses associated with these types of infections. You must learn to control the harmful germ-life that affect the wellness of your mouth, your body, and your unborn child, both *chemically* and *mechanically*.

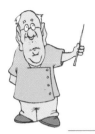
Dr. Paul H. Keyes advises, "You must disorganize, disperse, detoxify and disinfect the bacterial biofilms that colonize on the surfaces of the teeth."

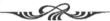

According to Dr. Keyes, "The therapeutic value of tooth brushing is attained not only by its potential to mechanically remove food particles and bacterial plaques, but also by its ability to deliver antibacterial agents to the surfaces of your teeth and gums which have not been adequately 'debugged' by the mechanical measures you have used."

So, from now on, I want you to think about self-care methods that will "de-bug" your teeth. From this new perspective, I am going to introduce you to **antibacterial oral hygiene** that will ensure excellent dental health.

This chapter is all about tooth brushing. Here you will learn the importance of brushing your teeth, the right way to brush your teeth, different types of brushes, and even how many different surfaces a tooth has. (The answer might surprise you!)

From the beginning, you may have been bombarded with a flurry of conflicting instructions on how to perform this vital ritual. Is it up and down? Side to side? Medium bristle? Hard? Soft? And … the biggest question of all: What in the heck is that little Hershey's Kiss-shaped thing on the end of the brush?

No matter how you learned to brush, the simple fact is that you should keep brushing. When it is properly done, the mechanical action of the brush interrupts the destructive process of the bacteria that not only cause damage to your teeth and gums but may also cause serious health problems in other parts of your body. We all know the *cosmetic* value of brushing. This chapter will emphasize the *therapeutic* value of brushing so that you will learn to disinfect rather than just clean. You can phase out your old way of thinking.

Who Taught Us How to Brush, Anyway?

I have probably seen almost as many styles of brushing teeth as I have seen patients throughout my thirty-plus years in dentistry. Yet, after all that time — and all those brushing methods — I always ask my patients to brush their teeth for me, no matter what their age.

I am always interested to see yet another variation on the theme. But I am hardly shocked at the ineffective techniques demonstrated by my new patients. Who ever taught us how to brush, anyhow? Was it our parents or siblings? Our teachers or friends? No one ever formally taught me. I was simply told to brush my teeth and make them look nice. As a result, I simply brushed my smile, — because that is all that showed!

Well, my parents never got a lesson either — so what did they know?

As the years progressed, however, I, like thousands of others, (close to 85% of the population, in fact) was developing gingivitis, the first stage of prolonged gum disease. If I hadn't gone to dental hygiene school in my early 20's, I would probably have been well on my way to losing my teeth like so many others in their 30's, 40's, and certainly 50's. After all, periodontitis is the major cause of adult tooth loss.

Fortunately for me, I learned how to brush properly in those intervening years. Now, I can pass along that knowledge to you.

A dear friend of mine gave me permission to print this poem he wrote to his son to encourage good brushing.

To Aaron, from Dad

It's getting late
So prance to the sink
To make your gums
A nice shade of pink.

Bedtime is near
Time to hush
Concentrate
And grab your brush.

Run the water,
Spread the paste
The Sandman's waiting
No time to waste.

Upstairs, downstairs
In and out
Around the tops
And all about.

Down your teeth
Across your gums
Wiggle that brush
Until it hums.

When your teeth
Are sparkling white,
Smile with pride
And kiss "Goodnight!"

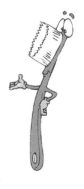

Marvin Steinberg

First Things First ... Holding the Brush

Pick up your toothbrush as if you were going to write your name with it. This is the "pencil grip," and it is a lot gentler on your teeth than holding your clenched fist around the brush— ouch! When you hold the brush with your entire fist around it, notice how you are using your upper arm and all its strength to scrub. When you hold the brush as you would hold a pencil, you use only the movements of your wrist, which are far less likely to be damaging. Think gentle. (From the way people brush, I can always tell those who have the cleanest kitchen floors!)

Pencil Grip

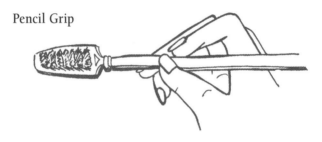

How to Brush

I want you to forget the concept of **tooth** brushing. Instead, be open to something new. Something unique. Something revolutionary. I want you to think about brushing your **gums**, not *instead* of brushing your teeth, but in *addition* to brushing your teeth.

The tiny space or crevice between your tooth and gums, the sulcus, is a fertile breeding ground for millions of *anaerobic bacteria*. Anaerobes live in an environment without oxygen, and are the same types of bacteria that live in deep puncture wounds. If these bacteria are allowed to grow into toxic plaques on the root surfaces, the gingival crevices enlarge and separate from the teeth. When these crevices, or *sulci*, become deeper than 1/8 inch, they are called pockets. These periodontal pockets are warm, dark, moist spaces without circulating oxygen, that are ideal hiding places for the anaerobes that are responsible for serious gum infections.

Now, watch yourself in the mirror. Holding your brush as you would a pencil, place it half on your tooth and half on your gums, slanting it toward the gum line at a 45° angle (see diagram, correct). At first, I want you to exaggerate the placement on your gums so you are actually more on your gums than on your teeth. Next move the brush back and forth in small scrubbing strokes no wider than the space of two teeth at a time.

Correct Angulation
45° angle towards gum line

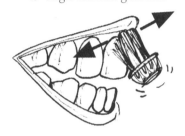

Incorrect Angulation
Flat against tooth

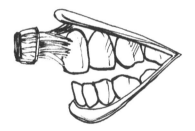

You can wiggle your toothbrush back and forth or do tiny circular movements — as long as the brush is aimed at the gum line and you are getting the bristles to go slightly under the gingival margin and in between your teeth. Dr. Lawrence Page of Temple University coined the term "root brushing" to describe this technique. Watch the difference between the correct angulation and simply placing the brush directly against your teeth (see diagram, incorrect).

You lightly scrub only two teeth at a time and count to six (one and two and three and four ...) before moving on to the next two teeth and repeating the process. If you have missing teeth, work around them and do the sides, or in betweens, for maximum tooth-to-brush exposure. When brushing your back teeth, hold the brush at the far end. This gives you more control and allows you to reach way in the back of your mouth without difficulty.

To brush the inside surfaces of your top and bottom front teeth, move the brush up and down rather than with the side-to-side motion you use for the rest of your teeth. Two full minutes of brushing is effective for contributing to the overall health of your teeth and gums.

Correct Tooth Brushing Method

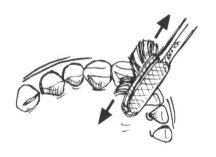   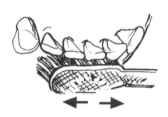

Upper Insides
Use an up and down stroke

Lower Front Teeth
Use a back and forth stroke

Again, your stroke should be very short, about the width of two teeth, back and forth, and "wiggly." Your brush should flex in and around the spaces and crevices where the anaerobic bacteria prefer to hide out. You should establish a routine, a specific order of brushing, so that you won't miss the same areas again and again. I always start on my upper left side, I brush all the outsides, all the insides, and then I move to the bottom left and follow the same pattern. Allow a full two minutes to cover all areas — top and bottom, inside and out.

This thorough technique accomplishes several things at once. It removes the bacterial biofilms along the gum line and somewhat in-between the teeth, massages your gums, and creates good circulation. This is important because gums, like muscles, need to be exercised and "toughened up." When the gums are stimulated, they become calloused, strong, and more resistant to injury and to the toxic by-products of the bacteria. They also exhibit a lighter pink color rather than the deeper reddish purple coloration of a person with a chronic periodontal condition. (Some mouths are more heavily pigmented and vary in color, however, just like your skin.) Just wait, after effective plaque control you will notice the difference in color in less than two weeks.

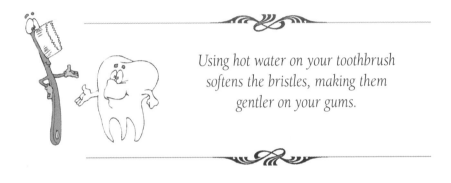

Using hot water on your toothbrush softens the bristles, making them gentler on your gums.

How often should you brush? Twice a day should be the *minimum*. Why? Simple. In the morning, brushing your teeth gets rid of the biofilms that have built up on your teeth overnight. Before bedtime is another vital period. When you sleep, your mouth and your teeth become more vulnerable to bacterial acids.

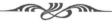

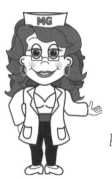

Brush as soon as possible after the last meal of the day, especially after eating or drinking anything with a high sugar or starch content. By keeping these residues at a very low level, you reduce the nutrients many plaque-forming bacteria depend on for their growth and survival, and minimize dental caries.

How Many Surfaces Are There on Each Tooth?

One day not so long ago, a new patient came into the office. She was middle-aged, very bright, and obviously quite successful in business. As I do with all my patients, I asked her, "How many surfaces do you think each tooth has?"

She thought briefly and answered triumphantly, "Two! An outside ... and an inside."

"OK" I replied. "There *are* two sides to your teeth — and then there are three more! The five surfaces of your teeth are: the outside of the tooth, number 1, the inside, number 2, the top side of the tooth, number 3 (also known as the 'biting surface'), and two sides, known as 'the in-betweens,' or proximal surfaces, number 4 and number 5. Every tooth has five surfaces and to be effective in your oral hygiene, **you must disinfect every surface of every tooth, every 24 hours.** That's my philosophy." So you see, no matter how impressive or successful someone is, I never take for granted that they automatically know the anatomy of the teeth, or how to sanitize them effectively. It is important to thoroughly decontaminate not only the outsides of your teeth, facing the cheeks, but the insides as well, facing the tongue. Also important to the health of your teeth are the biting or chewing surfaces, *and* the in-betweens, the interproximals.

How often?

Remember ... **Every** surface of **every** tooth, **every** 24 hours.

Obviously, if the teeth are close together, with no missing teeth, the bristles of a brush won't fit between them so you will need a different tool to sanitize surfaces 4 and 5. We will discuss those proximal surfaces later on.

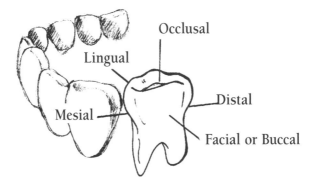

Five Tooth Surfaces

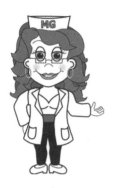

Let's Review:

To get the most out of your at-least-twice-daily brushing sessions, always remember to do the following:

- *Hold your toothbrush like a pencil.*
- *Place half of the brush on the tooth, half on the gum, and angle at 45-degrees toward the gum-line. Think gums!*
- *Brush with short, back and forth, scrubbing strokes (up and down on inside front teeth).*
- *Cover only two teeth at a time.*
- *Count to **six** — "one and two and three and ..." — as you scrub.*
- *Follow a routine: begin and end in the same place each time you brush.*
- *Use gentle pressure.*
- *Feel the bristles lightly massaging the gums and creating good circulation.*
- *Brush for a full two minutes.*

Congratulations! You are already well on your way to a healthier mouth, for both you and your baby. But, there's still much more to learn. We've covered "brushing," now let's move on to "Brushes."

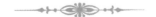

Manual Brushes

If you use a manual toothbrush, I recommend one with soft, rounded, nylon bristles. (Natural bristles are better than nylon only if you have acrylic bridgework — you will have to ask your dentist for a more personalized recommendation.)

A softer brush is always preferable to one with hard, stiff bristles. Consider using one that is smaller than what you are used to, as it is easier to manipulate around the often-cramped confines of your mouth. This is especially true if you have spaces caused by missing teeth, or if you have trouble reaching behind your hard-to-get-at back molars.

I also recommend that you alternate brushes, using several different brushes daily, as each brush will benefit from drying out between brushings. So, if you brush 3 times a day, you should have *three* toothbrushes. This is a good opportunity to try out different brushes, testing various brands, bristle lengths, and sizes, etc., to see which one you like best.

No matter which brush you choose, it is my personal opinion that all brushes should be replaced every two to three months, long before the bristles splay and shred, which is often caused by using too much pressure. I believe frayed or worn brushes, once they develop sharp edges, eventually become ineffective for brushing, though Dr. Keyes likes them for delivering medications (which I will talk about later).

You should also replace a brush after having a cold or a sore throat, because brushes will harbor bacteria and you can actually re-infect yourself from a germ-laden toothbrush. Ever notice that it seems to take forever to get rid of that nasty flu?

Well, it could just be your toothbrush!

And, by the way, NEVER share a toothbrush with anyone.

Electronic and Sonic Brushes

These relatively newfangled gadgets seem to be popping up in stores all over the country these days. They are brushes that electrically move vertically, horizontally, or even in combination.

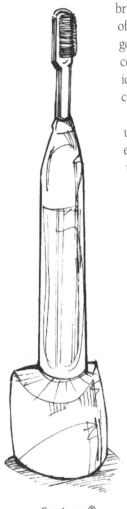

One of the newest technologies is the Sonic toothbrush, which is so advanced that it vibrates at thousands of vibrations per minute. This particular brush is very good at dislodging and disturbing the harmful bacterial colonies growing on your teeth and in the gingival crevices surrounding them, which, as we have learned, can cause gum infections.

There are many good choices, though I recommend using a toothbrush that feels good to you, that you will enjoy, that is practical for your particular budget, and that won't just sit there collecting dust next to your crocheted toilet paper cover because it's too difficult or frustrating to use.

Whichever model you decide to purchase, don't let technology take the place of what you have already learned. The method of brushing with either an electronic or sonic brush is *exactly* the same as using a manual toothbrush. (See *Review,* above.) The directions on the electronic/sonic brush may instruct you to "hold the brush stationary," but I don't think this method is very effective. After all, could you do a good job on your kitchen floor by just *holding* the mop against the surface?

Didn't think so ...

The Sonicare® even has an automatic timer that beeps every 30 seconds and shuts the brush off after two minutes. It is called a Quadpacer®

Sonicare®
Toothbrush

because 30 seconds is roughly the amount of time it should take to do one quarter of your mouth thoroughly.

But we're not done yet. There's another, often neglected area to address when you are brushing your teeth. What is it? You will find out in the next chapter.

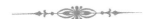

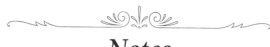

Notes

Chapter Three

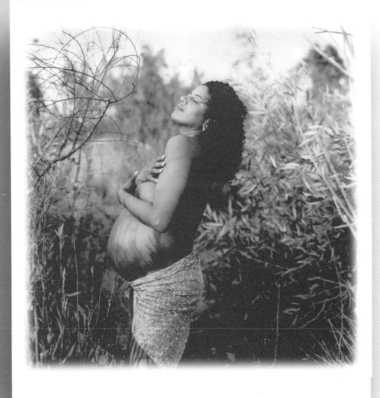

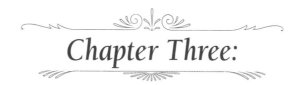

Chapter Three:

Bad Breath

ral malodor, known also as halitosis or bad breath, can result not only from infected teeth and gums but also from the tongue. Let's perform a quick experiment, one I've used with thousands of amazed patients in my chair over the years. Stick out your tongue right now. Look in the mirror, and notice the yellowish *film* on your tongue. Look way in the back. If you have *never* brushed your tongue, and chances are many of you haven't, the coating will tend to be quite heavy.

Now can you guess where bad breath comes from?

Everything that goes into your mouth — popcorn, ginger ale, pickles and ice cream, corn chips, cough drops, and all the exotic foods one craves during pregnancy — passes over your tongue. Inevitably, food residues and bacteria collect in the tiny grooves and spaces on your tongue and decompose there. Like decaying food in the refrigerator, this stuff eventually turns smelly and foul.

The guilty parties in yucky mouth odors are bacteria. Bacteria produce their natural by-products, and the results are nitrogenous, sulfuric toxins that cause what is known as "stinky breath." Therefore, to avoid this nasty side effect, your tongue must be cleansed regularly.

Daily is best ...

Offensive Bad Breath

Everyone has bad breath from time to time. Take that mouthwash commercial on TV that shows two lovers waking up in the morning, looking lovingly at each other for only an instant before covering their mouths, turning their heads, and muttering "good morning" without actually *breathing* in each other's face?

I'm not particularly concerned about morning breath, occasional bad breath from onions or garlic or other spicy foods, or even the habitually bad breath that results from regular smokers or coffee drinkers. What I am concerned about is offensive bad breath, the kind that comes from a nasty gum infection. The kind that smells like something is dying — right inside your mouth!

I can remember a particular patient who came into our office one day. My boss, the dentist, a very forthright person and also a committed teacher of dental and oral care, walked into the operatory where sat this woman and said, "Phew! I can smell your breath clear into the next room."

The woman broke down in tears and told him that no one had ever had the nerve to say that to her. Even though it was embarrassing and hurt her feelings to hear it spoken aloud like that, she was so grateful to him for having the guts to actually come right out and say it.

She had suspected for a long time that her bad breath was a problem, but simply didn't have the nerve to ask anyone to be honest with her and confirm what she had long feared. I could see her visibly relax as if a huge weight had been lifted off her shoulders, once the initial shock and shame of hearing the words out loud had passed.

She thought something was "stinky," and now she had confirmation. She was now ready to listen and get into treatment for what turned out to be a very advanced case of gum disease.

She was ready to move on ...

Are you?

Bad breath is not *just* about the infection. While that is certainly serious enough, for some people *halitosis*, or "bad breath," is a social problem that affects every aspect of relating to another person. It inhibits dating and socializing, and can even affect one in a work situation when having to talk up close with others, or even in applying for a job, or working your way up the corporate ladder — where image certainly is *everything.*

The prospect of kissing a spouse or a lover or a first date can be so fraught with anxiety that it inhibits one's desire to be close to another — for fear of offending them. Imagine being so ashamed of your breath that it might stop you from getting close to that very special someone?

There is so much anxiety about bad breath that the mouthwash industry in the United States alone, in the year 2002, sold $885 million dollars worth of oral rinses. Too bad that mouthwashes, rinses, sprays, and mints are only a temporary measure: like perfume sprayed over smelly armpits, mouthwashes are largely ineffective because they don't really get to the *source* of the problem.

What exactly is the problem? 80 to 90% of all bad breath comes from the mouth. On rare occasions, there are some other causes. A sweet, sickly smell is often associated with diabetes; an ammonia-like smell may be linked to kidney failure; and a fecal smell from the mouth, fortunately a rather rare occurrence, can indicate an intestinal blockage. A throat, sinus, or lung infection can also cause the foul breath.

Some people believe that bad breath originates from the stomach. That source is more unusual than you might think. The stomach is basically a closed system. The esophagus, which is the tube that connects the mouth to the stomach, is generally a one-way tube that remains "closed" a majority of the time. The exceptions are burping and vomiting, which are events that happen only occasionally and are not the source of chronic halitosis.

Before we explore the mouth for the various causes of bad breath, if you have any suspicion that you might have a case of halitosis, the following self-test is very revealing.

Take the Bad Breath Test:

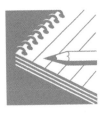

The following test is specifically designed to help you see if you qualify for the *Halitosis Hall of Fame:*

- Lick the back of your hand. Wait about 30 seconds, and then smell your hand. Is there a bad odor?

- Take a look at your gums. Are they red, swollen, or do they bleed when you brush or floss or when you press on them? Do you see pus or blood?

- Take a piece of dental floss, swipe and move your floss around several of your back teeth, top and bottom, and then smell the floss. That is what people smell when they are up close.

- Take a piece of gauze and run it over the top back portion of your tongue. Is the gauze yellowish? Smell it.

- Cup your hands in front of your mouth, exhale, and breathe in. This is what others smell when you talk to them.

- Has your dentist or hygienist told you that you have gum disease and should improve your oral hygiene? This is generally a good indicator that your breath may be giving off "warning signs."

- Now, for the *ultimate* test: If you are brave and you have a very good friend, ASK your friend. Tell her that you want to know the truth. Many people will not tell you because they don't want to hurt your feelings.

Let's explore the occasions on which your mouth may be the cause of bad breath. An abscessed tooth, a few cavities, a smelly denture, and chronic post-nasal drip are the "sometimes" culprits of bad mouth odor.

An abscess is an infection. It drains pus into the mouth and, as a result, smells putrid. Cavities are decayed tooth material. And we all know the various smells that result from decay. (Remember that meatloaf surprise you've had in the fridge for three weeks!?)

Dentures, usually made of acrylic, are porous and tend to absorb odors. The mucous of post-nasal drip rolls down the throat, where some of it falls onto the back of the tongue and hangs around for a while. In doing so, the bacteria start to break it down and, after a few days, the smell can get pretty foul.

Just as the tongue has many hiding places, the gums in periodontal infections are puffy, inflamed, and are pulled away from the sides of the teeth creating a "pocket" for bacteria to hide. These are very fertile breeding grounds for the anaerobes to do their thing — and cause stinky breath as a result.

It is easy to see how any — or *all* — of the above conditions could be a source of bad breath! But what else is there? Certain medications such as decongestants, antihistamines, antidepressants, certain antibiotics, and others can cause your mouth tissues to dry out. Smoking produces the same result.

During sleep, your mouth membranes also dry out due to the decrease in saliva flow. When oxygen in the mouth diminishes, an environment is created that nurtures the growth of anaerobic bacteria — those that cannot flourish in the presence of oxygen — whose by-products include Volatile Sulfur Compounds, and other noxious compounds, which in turn cause bad breath. These VSCs include methyl mercaptan and hydrogen sulfide (which smells like rotten eggs … remember that from chemistry lab?) and volatile fatty acids.

Your Tongue and Your Breath

You took a look in the mirror. Did your tongue have a white or yellowish coating on it? The thicker the layer, the longer it has been there and the more severe or chronic the malodor problem. Because the tongue contains tiny nooks, crannies, and fissures, there are plenty of ideal hiding places for the bacteria to flourish. There they produce the toxic, fetid compounds from the foods we eat, from bacterial waste products, and from the natural process of skin cells that are sloughed off in the course of daily living. If these and other malodorous blends are undisturbed or not "oxygenated," they will create the odor of chronic halitosis.

The Tongue (nooks and crannies)

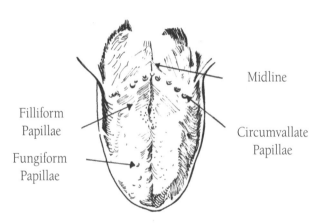

Midline

Filliform
Papillae

Circumvallate
Papillae

Fungiform
Papillae

In their article on "Assessing the Contribution of Anaerobic Microflora of the Tongue to Oral Malodor" for the *Journal of the American Dental Association*, E. H. De Boever and W. J. Loesche found that the tongue plays an important role in the production of "oral malodor."

While studying the role of tongue surface characteristics and oral bacteria in halitosis development, the authors studied a variety of possible sources for oral malodor. These included examining "odor measurements, volatile sulfur compound levels, periodontal parameters, tongue surface characteristics, presence of trypsin-like activity of organisms on the tongue and teeth and bacteriological parameters in 16 participants with complaints of oral malodor." They found that the "anaerobic bacteria residing on the tongue plays (sic) an essential role in the development of halitosis."

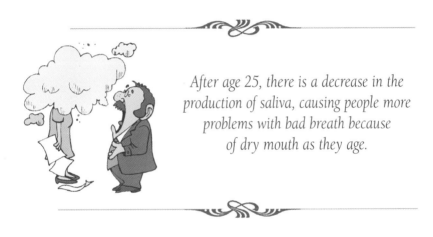

After age 25, there is a decrease in the production of saliva, causing people more problems with bad breath because of dry mouth as they age.

Certain essential oils have been found useful in the fight against bad breath. Clove oil, the smell that most reminds us of a dental office, has certain antibacterial qualities that are pleasant and soothing. Eucalyptus, mint, and cinnamon have also been used as breath deodorizers, but since most Westerners associate the clean smell and taste of mint with freshness, peppermint is one of the most popular additives to mouthwashes. Chewing on parsley, abundant in chlorophyll, has been used as a natural deodorizer in folk medicine for years.

However, these are mere stopgap measures and, for those with chronic halitosis, act much like putting a Band-Aid on a broken arm!

So what can we do to control this problem?
It is basically very simple.

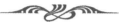

*We must eliminate the bad bacteria in our mouths
to ensure that they don't produce the foul smelling
compounds that result in chronic bad breath.*

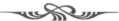

One easy and effective way to remove bacteria and debris from your tongue is with a specially designed tool, known in the industry as a "tongue scraper," which is sold in most department stores and pharmacies. I personally like to use a very small, soft toothbrush to cleanse my tongue. Other people use a small spoon, a dull knife, a tongue depressor, or even a Popsicle stick! You can be creative with your homemade tongue scraper, as long as you remember to be gentle.

As with your toothbrush, experiment until you find something you like. The tongue scraper is as simple to use as its name implies. Stick out your tongue, place the scraper as far back on your tongue as you can without gagging, and pull forward while pressing lightly.

During pregnancy your gag reflex is probably at its peak in the morning so you may want to choose another time of day, like evening or late afternoon, to scrape or brush your tongue. Be gentle yet firm. You never

Tongue Scraper

want to have your tongue bleed. This technique only takes seconds, yet it is invaluable for eliminating those bad breath germs from the surface of your tongue. You will enjoy a mouth that feels cleaner, tastes sweeter, and is definitely fresher than ever before.

Tongue scraper? Check. What's next? There are products on the market that replace saliva, or at least moisten the mouth if you frequently have the bad breath and other nagging symptoms of "dry mouth."

Information and Products for Your Breath

There is serious research and testing going on at this time by a dentist in Australia, Dr. Geoffrey Speiser, who is developing products for bad breath. His web site, www.breezecare.com, is educational, and quite interesting as well.

Meanwhile, any chemicals that cause an increase in oxygen, and an increase in the flow of saliva, are useful to inhibit the anaerobic bacteria that cause bad breath. These include hydrogen peroxide and chlorine dioxide. There are some others on the market that are worth the time to check out.

Another site comes from Israel and is run by Dr. Mel Rosenberg, professor of microbiology, Goldschleger School of Dental Medicine, Tel Aviv University. It has questions and answers addressing almost every concern you could have, along with a little humor: www.tau.ac.il/~melros/. The following comes directly from his web site: "According to ancient Jewish Law, if a man marries and finds out that the breath of his wife is offensive, that is grounds for divorce. He therefore has no obligation to fulfill the terms of his marriage contract."

Rowpar Pharmaceuticals have a valuable web site, www.smilekiss.com. They sell products containing chlorine dioxide that have been successful in eliminating VSCs. We have used them in our dental practice with great success, and most patients like them very much. I hope you will, too.

I also received some information and samples of another product called Therabreath® that can be found at: www.therabreath.com. They have a variety of rinses, nasal and oral sprays, chewing gum, and tooth gel that refresh your breath and taste. They are very happy to answer any questions about bad breath and oral health by email at info@drkatz.com.

You now have some excellent resources, products, and relevant information about the various unpleasant odors that come from your mouth, beneath and between your teeth, gums, and tongue. So, by utilizing this information, you will be prepared to meet and greet anyone, without worrying about offensive bad breath. Please note that web sites change frequently. Web addresses are accurate as of this writing.

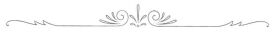

Notes

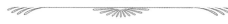

Chapter Four

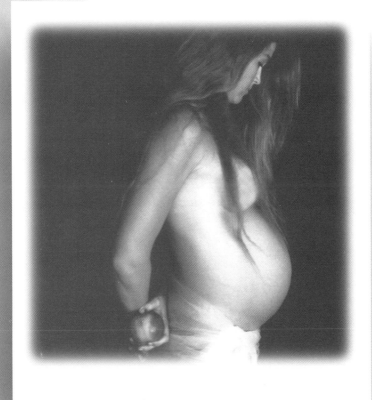

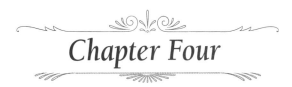

Chapter Four

Mama Gums' Magic Mix

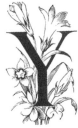

ou likely have a key to a cleaner, fresher, healthier mouth lying around the house right now. In fact, three of the most powerful ingredients that form your own chemical arsenal for fighting gum disease are far from mysterious. They are common household products you can probably find in your kitchen and/or bathroom this very minute: baking soda, salt, and hydrogen peroxide.

Used in combination just once a day as a homemade "toothpaste," these powerful chemicals have a devastating effect on the bacteria in the mouth that are responsible for gum disease. They are the antibacterial weaponry used to detoxify your mouth.

While doing research at the National Institutes for Health in the mid-1970s, Dr. Keyes made a startling discovery. He found that solutions of table salt (sodium chloride) and baking soda (sodium bicarbonate) kill on contact, many of the bacteria associated with periodontal infections. This explained why people who consistently used salt and soda as a dentifrice were less likely to have destructive periodontal disease. For many years Pycopay, a dentifrice that consisted of sodium bicarbonate (65%) and salt (35%), could be found in some drug stores.

Dr. Keyes, in addition to having some of his patients irrigate with a strong salt solution, had them brush their teeth with baking soda that was slightly moistened with hydrogen peroxide. This combination didn't really catch on until years later, when the toothpaste companies jumped onto the bandwagon when they realized how beneficial — not to mention *profitable* — this "magic mixture" could be. Unfortunately, as I will discuss later on in the book, *none* of the toothpastes available on the market today give us a high enough concentration of baking soda or peroxide to control bacterial growth.

In a letter he wrote to me, Dr. Keyes stated, "As an anti-infective mixture, the combination of sodium bicarbonate and hydrogen peroxide is hard to beat. Properly used, it will disorganize, disperse, detoxify, *and* disinfect the bacterial biofilms that colonize surfaces of the teeth."

This magical homemade paste can stop the progression of periodontal infection, and eliminate all of the following: bleeding, smelly breath, and tender, swollen tissues of the gum. It may even brighten your teeth a bit in the process. Best of all, you can begin using these chemicals right now to start making a noticeable difference in your total body health.

Baking Soda

Baking soda, also known as "sodium bicarbonate," has not only been an effective dentifrice but also a remedy for stomachache for many, many years. I can fondly remember my own grandmother mixing a tablespoon of the odorless white powder into a glass of water and drinking it, to cure an upset stomach.

I now understand why: It is an **excellent** acid neutralizer.

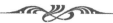

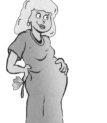 **A Special Precaution:** *If you are pregnant or wish to become so, or if you have high blood pressure or have been warned to eat a low-sodium diet, you must ask your doctor if it is appropriate for you to use baking soda and sea salt in your oral hygiene regime. It should be OK as long as you do not swallow it. Epsom salt may be an acceptable alternative.*

Baking soda is also a good cleaner, polisher, and deodorizer — not just in your refrigerator, but also in your mouth. As well as it performs as an antacid in the stomach, baking soda likewise will neutralize many bacterial toxins in your mouth. Microbial plaques or biofilms can be eliminated and controlled during the early stages of gingivitis. Baking soda makes an excellent antibacterial because when mixed with water and fully dissolved, it kills many disease-causing bacteria on contact and neutralizes their toxic by-products.

It is even more potent when mixed with peroxide, because the "fizzle" that results helps to disorganize and disperse microorganisms growing on tooth surfaces and in gingival crevices.

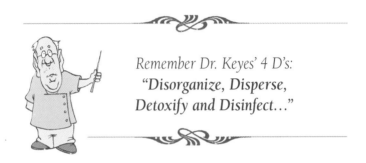

Remember Dr. Keyes' 4 D's:
"Disorganize, Disperse,
Detoxify and Disinfect..."

In 1988, Arm and Hammer first introduced a toothpaste containing baking soda as an over-the-counter version of Dr. Keyes' paste for the prevention and treatment of early gingivitis. This is also for people who have their infection under control and need a product for maintenance.

It will pay for you to shop skeptically. Many toothpastes, merely because it sounds good to include baking soda on the label, actually contain very small amounts. We know that the actual baking soda content needs to be relatively high (at least 65%) to be effective as an antibacterial.

For instance, Mentadent contains around 5% baking soda, and most other toothpastes contain anywhere from 1% to 20% — except Arm and Hammer, which has three different products ranging from about 35% - 95%. Arm and Hammer Dental Care® tooth powder, which is difficult to find, has the highest amount of baking soda, and is nearly as good as making your own — which of course is a full 100%!

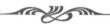

If the taste of the baking soda is offensive at first, you can coat the bristles of your toothbrush with a pleasant tasting toothpaste and then dip it into the baking soda. Brush with this until eventually you will get used to the taste of straight baking soda. I didn't like it at first but now I actually enjoy the fresh taste and the slippery-smooth feeling I have when I run my tongue over my teeth.

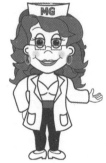

Toothbrushes can be placed in the dishwasher to sterilize them. "Germy" brushes have been shown to harbor and transmit bacteria and viruses, especially if you are using conventional toothpastes. "With baking soda, your toothbrush is kept quite clean, (microbiologically)," says Dr. Robert White of California. Another method of sanitizing your toothbrush is by dipping it in hydrogen peroxide and then into a mild Clorox solution.

Salt

Ordinary table salt, or sodium chloride, can be used very effectively as an ingredient of Mama Gums' *Magic Mix*, although I prefer the sea salt that can be found easily in health food stores, or even some grocery stores. Again, if you have high blood pressure, you may want to eliminate table salt as part of your own personal *Magic Mix*.

As I mentioned earlier, Epsom salt, otherwise known as magnesium sulfate, can be used instead of baking soda because it doesn't contain any sodium. But check with your doctor first.

Hydrogen Peroxide

Hydrogen peroxide, located on your grocery or drug store shelves in that familiar industrial brown bottle, is most commonly found in a 3% solution. Don't get sidetracked by the math. The percentage simply means that the bottle's contents are 97% water and 3% hydrogen peroxide.

This beneficial chemical is actually an *anti-infective agent* and was a staple in my medicine chest when my son was little. You have probably watched it foam and fizzle when you put it on a scraped knee or a deep cut. I have even used it on my cats when they got into a catfight!

The reason it effervesces is because it is loaded with oxygen (it is also a powerful oxidizer), which it releases in the presence of *catalase*, an enzyme found in blood, tissue cells, and bacterial by-products. As your mouth gets healthier, you will notice how much less the peroxide will foam when you use it.

This is a *good* thing ...

An interesting fact about hydrogen peroxide is that our bodies actually manufacture it in our cells to fight infection. In fact, it *must* be present for our immune system to function properly. One type of white blood cell, a neutrophil, actually kills invading bacteria by producing a deadly (to the bacteria, anyway) combination of enzymes, hydrogen peroxide, and other chemicals.

Where there are a lot of bacteria present in a particular area, such as an infection in your mouth, "pus" will form. This pus is actually dead white blood cells and other cellular debris. Using the phase contrast microscope, we see evidence of these pus cells clumped together and in large numbers.

Mama Gums' Magic Mix

The easiest way to make *Magic Mix* is to get yourself a small container with a cover, into which you will place a half cup of baking soda (sodium bicarbonate) with a teaspoon of salt. If you don't have any measuring devices, don't worry. This mixture has a lot of room for error. Don't fret if the proportions are not exact.

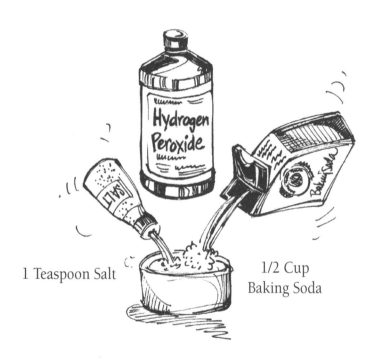

1 Teaspoon Salt

1/2 Cup
Baking Soda

These two initial ingredients should be mixed together to form a white powder. Next, wet your toothbrush with hydrogen peroxide — a quick dunk will do (I use the cap of the peroxide bottle) — and then dip your brush into the container of powder. It should stick quite well, and a generous amount is what you need to disinfect your whole mouth in one simple process. (If you prefer, you can put the peroxide in a small glass, add a little pleasant-tasting mouthwash if you wish it flavored, then dip into the powder.)

Remember: One dunk. One dip. Now you've got *Magic Mix!*

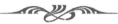

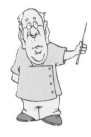

*Dr. Paul Keyes quips that one should use a "truckload" of baking soda. Dr. Robert White recommends using 10 brushes full per session of tooth brushing. You can use anywhere between one **very generous** dip and a truckload, and I know you will notice a difference.*

Also remember: If your gums become tender or irritated, you may have to discontinue the peroxide for a few days. Then go back to it, diluting it with half water, or even three quarters water, (a little mouthwash is fine, too) and make a solution that has just a little bit of peroxide.

It is **definitely** the peroxide, and not the baking soda, that can make your mouth tender. I suggest starting out with diluted peroxide first, and then gradually working up to the full strength version as your mouth gets used to this beneficial chemical. In any event, you should never be using more than the 3% solution of peroxide anyway.

This *Magic Mix* is to be used once a day, and *only* once a day, not more often. Most of us think "more is better," but if we do this process more frequently than once every twenty-four hours, our gums can become quite sore. This will defeat the purpose of using *Magic Mix* and even set you back a few days in your regimen because your gums will be too tender to even brush properly.

If you have pregnancy gingivitis and you are already sore, try some Glyoxide® for a couple of days before using *Magic Mix*, and then begin with diluted peroxide.

Coupling your brushing techniques with Mama Gums' *Magic Mix* produces positive, visible results within ten short days. If before starting this process your gums had been bleeding when you brushed or flossed, you will be happy to see the bleeding diminish within a week or so.

You will also notice a change in the color of your gum tissue, from a deep color to a paler shade, and your gums will become less "shiny." Eventually, as you get even healthier, your gums will have a "stippled" appearance, much like the skin of an orange.

Remember, you are not just decontaminating your teeth and gums. You are controlling infections in your mouth that affect your whole body's health, contributing to a healthier pregnancy, and a healthier baby as well. Keep the process up, and your mouth will truly start to feel the *Magic!*

So will the rest of you ...

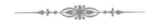

Chapter Five

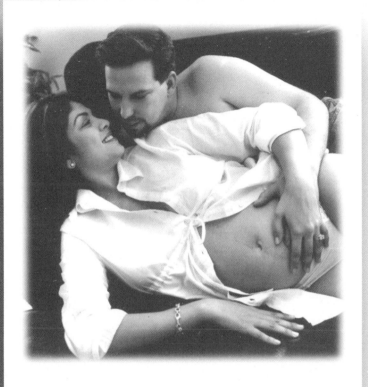

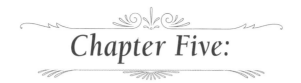

Chapter Five:

Flossing

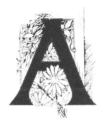patient once asked me this question, "Do I really have to floss my teeth?"

"No," I answered, "only the ones you want to keep."

This usually gets a laugh, possibly because it hits so close to home for most of us, but to properly decontaminate your mouth and rid yourself of the bacterial bad guys, you must remove them from the in-between surfaces of your teeth, surfaces 4 and 5.

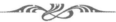

Remember, disinfect every surface of every tooth every 24 hours.

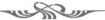

Along with tooth brushing, flossing has been the mainstay of most dentists' recommended home care routine. Flossing once a day, they say, is essential to remove the bacterial plaque from areas in between the teeth that your toothbrush can't reach. *Flossing is preventative, not curative, in that it removes the biofilm **before** it can do damage, but does nothing to affect an existing infection.*

As important as dentists tell us flossing is, surveys show that as many as 80% of us don't floss at all. Moreover, of the 20% who do floss, albeit irregularly, most don't do it properly. Ineffective flossing will leave bacteria in place to breed and do damage; in some cases, flossing incorrectly can actually force bacteria below the gum line, and sometimes cut the gums, opening entryways for the microscopic invaders.

My position on flossing is: Take the time to learn to do it correctly, and then do it.

Which Floss Shall I Use?

The floss you use is a matter of personal preference, which you will only discover through trial and error. There are ever-growing numbers of floss options: waxed or unwaxed; flavored or unflavored; fluoride-impregnated; baking powder-coated; silk or nylon; or ribbon tape. The thickness of the floss is a consideration when it comes to getting it between your teeth.

Very thin floss can be sharp and can cut the gums. The taste may make it more or less pleasant. Waxed floss slides more easily between tight teeth; unwaxed floss squeaks against the tooth to tell you when it is clean, but shreds more easily. Your choice of floss can make it fun — or dishearten you. Pick one that feels good, and that you find easy and comfortable to use. I personally like Glide® made by Gore. It's more comfy for both your fingers and your gums and it doesn't fray.

I once worked for two outstanding periodontists. One was adamant about the use of *unwaxed dental floss*, saying that the waxed type was sticky and would leave a residue on the teeth that would attract plaque. The other one recommended only *waxed dental tape*; he thought the waxed gentler on the tissue and he liked the broader surface area of the tape vs. the narrow string.

Each was committed to his own point of view.

Personally, I prefer that you experiment with several different brands and determine for yourself which one you like. My opinion is — it doesn't matter! The "best" one will be the one you are likely to use.

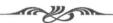

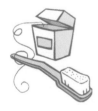

A Special Precaution: Flossing should not be used as a routine to remove food that is constantly being impacted between your teeth. This is most likely a defect that needs dental attention.

How Do I Floss?

Having chosen your floss, here is the right way to use it. Pull out about 18 inches. Wrap most of it (not too tight! — no cutting off circulation) around one middle finger, the rest around the middle finger of the other hand, and leave two or three inches held between your thumb and forefinger. Holding the floss taut, work it gently back and forth (like a shoe-shine motion) and into the space between your teeth. Don't let it snap onto your gums, as this can cut the skin.

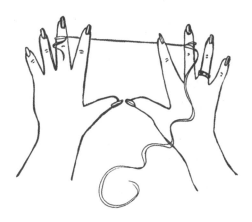

Curve the floss around the tooth, forming a C-shape at the gum line, and move it up and down several times against the tooth, (never against the gums) scraping away the particles and plaque. Work it into the space between the tooth and gum only as far as it will comfortably go. Wind on to a new piece of floss after each tooth. Keep going until you finish all your teeth. (If you run out of floss, pull more off next time; I use about a full arm's length — fingertips to chin — per flossing.) Make sure you do the "behind" of the last tooth.

Keep practicing. The important thing is to *do* it. Don't worry about doing it absolutely right the first few times. Don't be discouraged if it takes you a dozen tries before you get the hang of it. It takes time to become an expert.

Holding The Floss

Flossing Upper Teeth
Form a "C" Shape with the dental floss around the tooth

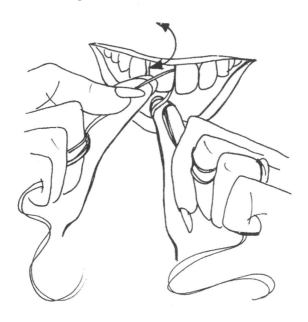

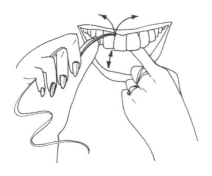

Flossing

- Gently "shoe-shine" the floss between the teeth

- Curve around the tooth "C" Shape

- Scrape up and down

- Rub against tooth, never against gum

Flossing Lower Teeth
Form a "C" Shape with the dental floss around the tooth

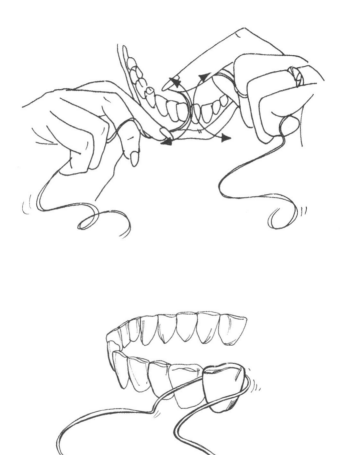

Shoe-shine behind the last tooth

Floss Accessories

There are a number of accessories available for those with "difficult" mouths or large fingers:

- **Floss threaders** are thin plastic loops that can get you into the tight spaces under and around bridgework, implants, and braces.

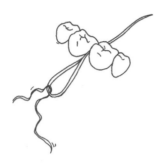

- **Dental Floss holders** come in many forms and are for those with compromised dexterity or large hands. This floss gadget can be a godsend. Just make sure that you move your wrist in such a way as to

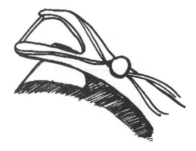

enable you to wrap the floss around the sides of the tooth, not just the space in between. Glide® disposable FlossPicks make flossing easy even between tight contacts.

- **Electric flossers**, a favorite for some patients, make flossing an easy, one-handed operation.

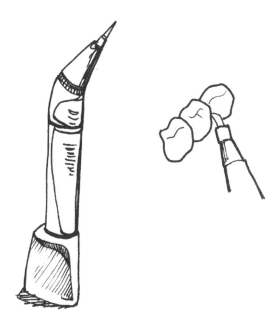

Use whatever product is easiest for you. The important thing is to hit those plaquey deposits once every 24 hours to keep the bacteria from getting a chance to recover and repopulate. They are prolific little critters (according to Dr. Loesche, some species double in number every 4.6 hours) and they will soon "get busy" all over again. Be ready to *disturb* them mechanically and attack them chemically every single day.

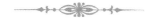

Notes

Chapter Six

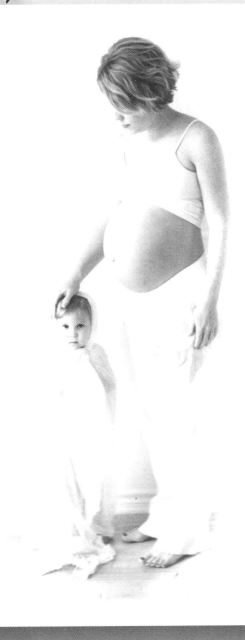

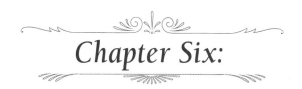

Chapter Six:

Irrigators and Solutions

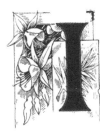n an ideal world, we dental professionals would have our patients so compliant and cooperative that every single one of them would brush three times a day, floss at least once a day, and come in every three months for their periodontal maintenance (recall) visit. Unfortunately, life just doesn't quite seem to happen that way. The reality is that patients often come in just once or twice a year for their "quick fix" and even those who are fully compliant can still harbor periodontal diseases that increase in severity over time.

I was shocked to learn that as few as 5% to 10% of the population in America actually floss their teeth on a *daily* basis — even after years of Johnson & Johnson telling people the wonderful results that can be had by flossing every day.

For those of you who simply hate flossing, aren't good at it, find it awkward or clumsy, simply just don't want to take the time, or best yet, just hate turning your fingers blue from the constriction of the nylon thread wrapped tightly around them, I have some good news. There *is* an alternative.

It's called **Irrigation**. Irrigation is a *mechanical* as well as a *chemical* process that enables you to dilute, disperse, and eradicate the harmful germ-life from your teeth and gums.

What is Irrigation?

Very simply, dental irrigation uses an electrical device to force a pulsating jet of warm water in a slim stream into the spaces between the teeth and gums; kind of like a water park for your mouth!

There is a basin into which you can place a variety of anti-infective medications, potent germ killers, that enable you to kill the bacteria lurking between your teeth and gums. We will discuss those medications a little farther along, and I'm sure you'll find one of them to your personal taste.

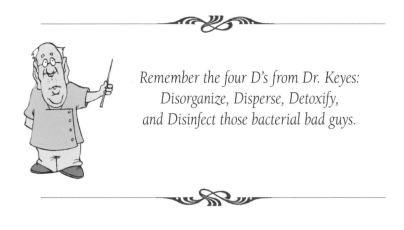

*Remember the four D's from Dr. Keyes:
Disorganize, Disperse, Detoxify,
and Disinfect those bacterial bad guys.*

This technique flushes food debris and plaque from your mouth, and chemically inhibits the germs that cause gum disease by reaching them where the common toothbrush and other dental tools don't, or can't, go. To be most effective, you should irrigate once or preferably twice a day.

While the manual toothbrush cleans to a depth of only around 1/8th of an inch below the gums, the irrigator, when combined with special tips, not only disrupts the surface bacteria, but also their toxic byproducts below the gum line to about a quarter of an inch. This process kills the sub-gingival bacteria and flushes them out from spaces other tools can't reach. (Special slim tips for deeper pockets can be obtained through the company that sells the irrigator.)

If you have never tried this wonderful tool, or even if you did years ago, and didn't quite get it right the first time, I strongly recommend that you do so. Or, try again, especially if flossing is not one of your favorite "hobbies." Irrigation is quite simple to do and very gratifying, as you can literally see bits and pieces of food and debris spilling into the sink at a surprising rate, even after brushing rather conscientiously.

In addition to the smorgasbord flooding out of your mouth, imagine all of the microscopic "stuff" that you are removing that you *can't* see. It is truly amazing to see how much "junk" can remain lodged between your teeth and gums, and discover how long it can remain there, only to be removed in one squirting session by the dental equivalent of a miniature fire hose!

If used correctly, the dental irrigator is a safe tool that not only cleans the in-between areas of your teeth and gums, but also has other advantages.

Irrigation:

- *Diminishes the numbers of bacteria and their by-products by diluting them and flushing them out of your mouth.*

- *Reduces inflammation and bleeding.*

- *Massages and toughens up the gum tissue.*

- *Flushes around orthodontic bands, brackets, and wires (braces), as well as crowns and bridgework.*

- *Reduces bad breath.*

- *Delivers antibacterial medications in hard-to-reach areas, such as under the gum line.*

- *Helps firm up your gums, enabling them to hug your teeth more tightly.*

- *Washes out food particles and toxins.*

- *Feels great!*

Irrigators are easy to use and very effective in preventing disease, as well as in maintaining a healthy mouth. I am recommending them more and more to children because irrigation is so much easier and much more fun than flossing. It is also wonderful for kids with braces. Many companies offer different colored, interchangeable tips, allowing family members to share this device.

A Special Note: Dental Irrigation is an *essential* part of periodontal therapy and should be part of your daily routine, especially during pregnancy.

How do I Use This Fancy Thingamajig?

First of all, a warning from Mama Gums: Until you get the hang of it, the irrigator *can* be quite messy. I use mine at my kitchen sink, not only because I have more space there than in my bathroom, but also because it is easier to clean up any unsightly "splatters."

Mama Gums Advises: Before you start, especially if your mouth is badly infected, I recommend rinsing first with an antibacterial mouthwash, such as Listerine® or Therasol®. A saturated solution of salt water or baking soda water works well, too. You can make that by taking several tablespoons of either salt or baking soda and stirring it into an 8 oz. glass of water. This simple step reduces the potency of the bacteria already present in your mouth, which could conceivably enter your bloodstream. It is precautionary and always a good, practical step before you do anything in your mouth that might cause bleeding.

Start by studying the diagram pictured here, perhaps keeping it directly in front of you as you position the tip the way it is illustrated in the drawing.

When you're comfortable with the diagram and the heft and feel of the irrigator itself, take the next step by watching yourself in the mirror. Begin by practicing moving the tip around and through your teeth at the correct angle, *without* water.

First Pass

When you do it for real, you will make two passes around your entire mouth with the irrigator. The first pass is at right angles to your teeth. That allows you to flush surface debris from your teeth and gums. On the second pass around your mouth, direct the water jet into the gingival crevices, those spaces between the teeth and gums.

Second Pass

Watch your movements and note how it feels. You will not be able to look in the mirror when you do it for real, because if you lift your head up, you will create an unbelievable mess, with water — and bits of food and other debris — shooting everywhere. (Kind of like spraying the mirror with a squirt gun!) Also, remember to keep your elbow raised slightly so that the water will trickle down into the sink rather than flooding your counter or sink tops.

As you can see, irrigating correctly relies on your sense of "feel." Keeping your head bent over the sink precludes the use of a mirror. Don't worry; soon you will get to know the nooks and crannies of your mouth on a more intimate basis. This is a good thing. We should all get to know our mouths better, and irrigation is one great place to start! I suggest that you begin with a few dry runs first before turning the machine on.

Now you're ready to do it for real. First, put the irrigator at its lowest pressure setting. Lean your head over the sink, and place the nozzle inside your mouth. Close your lips loosely around the tip of the nozzle, leaving a slight gap for the water to run out, and *then* turn it on.

Next, move the nozzle along your gum line at a right angle, that is, parallel to the biting surfaces of your teeth. To get the most benefit from this experience, make sure that you hesitate between each and every tooth for at least a couple of seconds. (See diagram below for a visual aid)

Warning: Never, ever, direct the flow of water down toward your gums the first time around. The objective is to go around your whole mouth the first time at right angles, concentrating on getting rid of the surface bacteria and debris first. If your mouth is badly infected and you don't do this preliminary step, you can possibly force bacteria and food debris into the gums and potentially

Lower Teeth Facials
(Outsides)
Right Angles (First Pass)

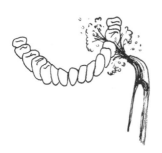

Lower Linguals (Insides)

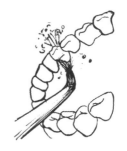

Upper Linguals
(Insides)

cause a condition known as *bacteremia*, where the bad organisms could enter your bloodstream and potentially cause you to get very sick or even die. I don't want you to be afraid to do this entirely beneficial procedure, but at the same time I want you to have a healthy respect for this wonderful piece of equipment and know that it will help get you healthy if used properly, but *could* make you sick if used *carelessly.*

You may now open your mouth and let the water continuously flow out into the sink. As you do so, you will begin to feel a glorious sense of accomplishment as you see the little crumbs of food, etc., pour out from the interdental nooks and crannies.

After you've gone once around your mouth thoroughly, repeat the process, this time with the tip directed into the sulcus. This will flush out the bacterial colonies while depositing the medication from your basin deep below the gum line where it will do the most good. It is the same type of lavage that doctors use in debriding a wound.

As your gums get healthier within the next two to four weeks, and you notice no bleeding, you can increase the water pressure to medium/high. I do not recommend using the irrigator on the highest setting at any time.

This whole process shouldn't take more than a few minutes to accomplish and, once you get used to it, you will find irrigation a lot easier than flossing. It doesn't require much dexterity to irrigate, and you don't need to open as wide as you must to manipulate floss around your teeth with tiny fingers or special gadgets.

Don't get me wrong. I am certainly not saying that I wouldn't be happy if you practiced both flossing *and* irrigating. And, ideally, I see irrigating as an adjunct to brushing and flossing, even though earlier I said it was merely an alternative. The exception is for those of you who would do neither, if left up to your own devices. The fact that the irrigator has the potential to deliver potent, anti-microbial solutions that are deadly to the bacteria between your teeth and gums is a tremendous plus! Once again, we are using **mechanical** means as well as **antibacterial** (chemical) warfare in the ongoing battle for your healthy mouth!

If you think about it, it's the home version of your hygienist's "rinse and spit," just with a little gusto added! Your mouth should now feel lighter and cleaner and I hope that you become positively addicted, as I am, to this altogether healthy feeling.

Simply seeing the sheer quantity of food debris that rushes from your mouth should keep you running back to the irrigator day after day, if only to rid yourself of the daily accumulation of our modern American way of eating.

Types of Irrigators

As with most "tools of the tooth trade," there are several different types of worthwhile irrigators on the market today from which to choose. Some are pricier than others, but all are effective. I will describe them below. Naturally you will want to inspect the devices for yourself before choosing the one you like.

Let's begin with that old reliable Water Pik®:

Water Pik®

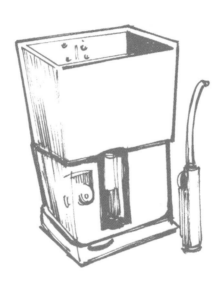

The first water irrigator invented was the **Water Pik®**. In fact, I can remember it being around when I was a young adult. However, this versatile and progressive periodontal product hasn't been content to sit around and rest on its laurels. In fact, it now has a new tip called a "Pik Pocket" that is superb at flushing out hard-to-reach areas. With a nod toward the sensitive nature of irrigating your own teeth, the Pik Pocket has a tiny rubber tip that helps prevent injury to your delicate gum tissues. It is said that this tip may possibly reach down as far as 7mm, although I do not have the data to support this claim.

There are several types of Water Pik® available these days, including a travel model, which makes it easy to do your self-care while on the road. The drawback is that with this model, it is best to use just warm tap water. The least expensive Water Pik® and the travel model are not recommended for use with salt or baking soda. Water Pik's professional model has an attachment to reach into deeper areas.

Hydro Floss®

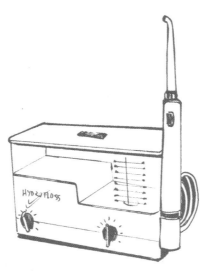

The Hydro Floss machine is a newer addition to the market of irrigators, and it has some special benefits to consider. The Hydro Floss device actually ionizes the water with small magnets in the hand piece, which reduces the ability of plaque to adhere to the teeth.

According to Dr. Dan Watt, co-founder of the *International Dental Health Foundation,* "Along with brushing and flossing, Hydrofloss irrigation provides the most cost effective, efficient mechanism for eliminating ... pathogenic biofilm."

In one study, Hydrofloss® was rated 3.07 on a scale of 1-4 and got a "good" or "excellent" rating from 83 percent of the clinical evaluators. Like the Pik Pocket, narrow tips are available that allow you to penetrate effectively deep below the gum line.

The price is considerably higher than the standard Water Pik®, which may be a consideration when weighing your irrigation options.

Viajet®

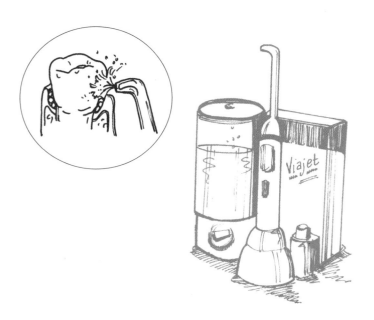

The Viajet Pro® is a reasonably-priced irrigator with convenient features and an attractive, redesigned look. It flushes food and debris above and below the gums and has an ultra-slim tip available to deliver solutions to the base of periodontal pockets. It is easy to adjust the stream of water and is gentle for tender gums. The SulcaSoft® tip, the latest product from Oratec, is a soft, tapered, and flexible tip that is very "patient friendly."

Panasonic EW176®

If you travel a lot, you will enjoy this battery-operated portable irrigator that really packs a wallop for its tiny size. Personally, I think this is a great one for kids who are too young or too unskilled to clean their teeth well. This is a nice tool to introduce them to irrigation. This irrigator is designed to irrigate selected areas rather than a full mouth, and can be ordered through **Oratec** at: 1-800-368-3529 or www.oratec.net.

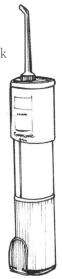

Perioflex® and Pocket Care®

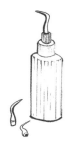

These are two small pocket or purse size versions that are used to irrigate specific sites in your mouth. They hold 2 ounces and ½ ounce respectively, and can also be ordered through Oratec.

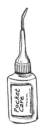

Regardless of price, brand name, basin size, portability, or popularity, the way I see it, it is vital to irrigate, period. Irrigation is a very valuable tool, no matter which irrigator you choose.

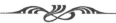

*A **Special Precaution:** If you have mitral valve prolapse or a heart murmur, you will want to consult your dentist regarding the benefits of irrigation or any new vigorous oral hygiene program. If you have a serious infection, your health professional may recommend starting an antibiotic to protect your heart, because heart valves are vulnerable to infection by the bacteria in the mouth. As gum disease progresses, bacteria can get into the bloodstream and even lodge on the heart valve. Even plain old **chewing** or simple **tooth brushing** in a mouth troubled with open wounds such as periodontal disease will spread bacteria into the bloodstream.*

Make sure that you maintain your irrigator by drying it out thoroughly between uses and NEVER add salt or baking soda directly into the basin, as the tiny crystals these products contain will eventually clog up the mechanism of the machine and render it useless.

Instead, always mix the solution in a glass and *then* pour the liquid into the basin, avoiding any undissolved crystals so that your machine will enjoy a long, productive life. *Flushing* your irrigator with very warm water after each use will add to its long lifetime. A drop or two of liquid detergent added to the flush every few weeks will make it last even longer.

Irrigating Solutions

Whatever type of irrigating tool you choose, if you want to be even *more* effective, you can add the mouthwash or chemicals of your choice. You can even use flavorings like mint or raspberry, etc. Since basin sizes vary, I am giving you measurements for each cup (8 oz.) of warm water.

- **Plain warm tap water** ... use it if there is nothing else available. It works fine and it will disorganize, dilute, and reduce bacteria by 50%.

- **Baking soda** ... two tablespoons in one of cup warm water. This is actually four times more effective than regular table salt. It is not easily absorbed through the tissues of the mouth and if you don't swallow it, it is okay for salt restricted diets. Be sure to flush irrigator.

- **Table salt** ... one to two tablespoons in one cup of warm water (again, mix in a glass first, then pour into irrigator basin because the salt crystals may clog your irrigator). This will dehydrate the bacteria and kill them. Be sure to flush irrigator thoroughly to eliminate salt water throughout tubing.

- **Hydrogen Peroxide** ... two capfuls in one cup of warm water. Although it is more often used in combination with baking soda and made into a toothpaste (introduced by Dr. Keyes in the 1970's), I have had patients use it in their irrigators with success. Please be aware that it can degrade the tubing of the irrigator.

- **OraChlor®** ... recommended by Dr. Paul H. Keyes in the 1980's. The active agent is Chloramine T, chemically similar to Chlorhexidine. It is 4 times more bactericidal than household bleach. Unfortunately, the taste, plus the fact that with frequent use it creates brown stains on your teeth, may make it unpleasant for home use. I used to have patients use it in the 1990's because it is very inexpensive and stable in its powder form. Once mixed with water, it will last 1-2 weeks. Confirm with your doctor that this is okay during pregnancy. Read him the label before you use it.

- **Povidine Iodine** ... (10% solution) can be bought over-the-counter and mixed with water or peroxide. This is one of my personal favorites. (I use it during treatment, mixed 50/50 with hydrogen peroxide, and apply it on the gums with a cotton swab.) Two capfuls per cup of warm water is antibacterial and effective. Please be careful not to get it on your clothing, because it stains. Taste is not too unpleasant diluted to this concentration. Not to be used if you are sensitive to iodine or shellfish.

- **Therasol®** ... My top favorite. Approximately one to two oz. per cup of warm water. It is pleasant tasting and highly effective, not only killing most bacteria but also yeasts and fungi. It is a broad-spectrum anti-microbial and is "chemically sticky," meaning that it doesn't wash off quickly like other solutions. It is gentle on your irrigator and will not clog the tubing. Unlike Chlorhexidine and OraChlor, it does not stain teeth or produce calculus. I like this product and use it in treatment as well as for my own personal use. Outside of its expense (about 62 cents per oz. in the small bottles), this is a very desirable product and can be bought in its concentrated form in ½ gallon size to make it more affordable (about 25 cents per oz.) Contact **Oratec** at (800) 368-3529 and say, "Mama Gums sent me..."

- **Peridex®** or **Chlorhexidine®** ... is probably the best-known antibacterial solution in the dental profession. They have been doing research on this mouthwash for over thirty years. It is sold by prescription as Peridex® and Periogard® in its .12% concentration. It is expensive. We made it available in our dental office at double that concentration. (.24% CHX.) Unfortunately, it does have some unpleasant side effects. If used on a daily basis, it produces dark brown stains on the teeth and increases hard deposits on the teeth in about 40% of users. The taste, although much improved over the original, is still mildly unpleasant and some people are affected by a temporary change in their taste receptors (20 minutes or so) making it advisable to go to that fancy restaurant before the irrigating experience. I have recommended it as a rinse, used full strength; as an application with a cotton swab in a specific area to minimize staining; and in the irrigator, one to two ounces per cup of warm water. In recent studies by Stavholz, it was found to be less effective in bleeding areas as it chemically binds to blood.

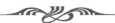

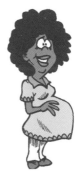

A Special Precaution: The effects of Peridex®during pregnancy have not been adequately researched. If you are pregnant or plan to become pregnant, check with your doctor and ask if it is okay for you to use this product, and all the others, to be absolutely safe.

Choosing one of the above solutions is not a decision to take lightly. Although all these solutions are effective, none of them are ideal. You must weigh the pros and cons of each one for yourself. Some stain the teeth, others taste awful, and some are actually toxic if swallowed. Because of these negative side effects, people often give up prematurely on irrigation altogether, much too early to see the positive benefits of these solutions.

If you think of these solutions as "medicine," and remember that most medicines don't taste very good but are nonetheless good for you and help you get healthy, you will be able to stick to it and gain the long-term benefits of these beneficial chemicals.

Although there may be no scientific basis for this recommendation, I like alternating my antiseptic solutions (i.e. I use bicarbonate of soda one week, then Chlorhexidine, then Therasol). After all, isn't variety the spice of life?

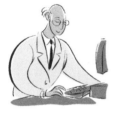 *Dr. Jorgen Slots says, "Local antibiotic therapy (delivered through an irrigator) can deliver sub-gingival doses about 100-fold higher than those possible by systemic therapy." Furthermore, "irrigation allows the use of antibacterial agents that cannot be given internally. Irrigators are particularly useful for people who have stomach sensitivity, or women who develop yeast infections when taking a prescribed course of systemic antibiotics. Also, for a person with only a few areas of infection in their mouth, the use of a systemic would be considered overkill."*

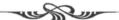

Herbs and essential oils have also been found to kill microorganisms, reduce inflammation, and even rebuild damaged tissue. Unfortunately, the FDA does not regulate these products and there is little research to validate their effectiveness. Since herbs used during pregnancy are very controversial, I have decided to omit them, but you can always contact a specialist who can give you guidance as to which herbs are appropriate for you. There are several companies that make natural toothpastes and powders from herbs, which you can check out on the Internet.

Is Rinsing Effective?

Rinsing is **not** irrigating. Rinsing, or swishing mouthwash around in your mouth for 30 or so seconds, is *inadequate* to do much of anything except make your breath fresher for a few minutes. (Maybe just long enough to get a kiss.) Rinsing does not deliver chemicals under your gum line by more than ½ a millimeter, which is not much at all. Most rinses are considered cosmetic (the ones that are sold over-the-counter), while only a few are therapeutic (the ones found in health food and medical supply stores).

The mouthwashes that contain high amounts of alcohol (18-26%) can actually make your tissues dry out, and cause a burning sensation on your tongue and cheeks. They may even result in *sloughing* of the mucous membranes of the cheeks. Some evidence even indicates that mouthwash with high alcohol content increases the risk for oral cancer. In addition, there are studies that suggest that smokers and people who drink alcohol tend to use mouthwash more frequently, linking the three most threatening oral cancer risk factors together. With daily use of a harsh and irritating rinse, you may even experience a "black, hairy tongue."

While this may sound like Hollywood's answer to the scariest horror movie ever, this condition is actually an enlargement of the taste buds on the surface of the tongue, resembling hair.

Note: If you *are* using a rinse for bad breath, those that I listed in the chapter on bad breath are helpful.

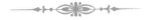

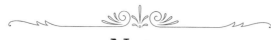

Notes

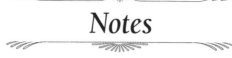

Chapter Seven

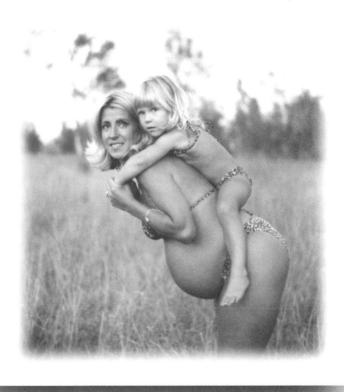

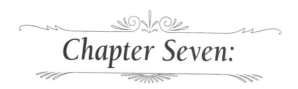

Chapter Seven:

Picks & Probes (and In-Betweens)

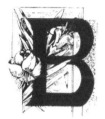

By now we should all know that using a toothbrush on only the "surfaces that show" is not enough to do an effective job in removing the bacterial biofilms that collect around your teeth and gums. We have to be creative to find gizmos and gadgets to remove the films from the proximal areas.

Dental floss, although very effective as a mechanical tool above the gum line, isn't easy to use on a regular basis. There have been many inventive ideas on how to accomplish removing the bacteria from what I call the "nooks and crannies." Remember always to be gentle. Here are a few tools that you will find helpful:

- **Rubber tip stimulators** are excellent for massaging your gums. (So now you know what that little Hershey's Kiss-shaped thing is on the end of your toothbrush.) It is a wonderful tool to work the baking soda and peroxide mixture under the gums. This delivery system is every bit as good as using a toothbrush, and I recommend it highly.

- **Toothpicks** are perfect for removing plaques and food debris from the in-between areas after lunch, and particularly useful if you are trying to quit smoking; they will give you something positive to do with your hands and keep your mouth busy. Work gently and be careful you don't poke yourself and cause bleeding.

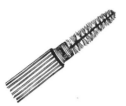

• **Interproximal brushes** are great for those large spaces between your teeth where chunks of food and bacteria hide out. They come with replaceable tips that are cylindrical or cone-shaped.

One of my favorites, the end-tuft brush made by Butler, has small, tapered nylon bristles just at the tip of the brush. It is perfect for cleaning behind the last molars as well as the awkward spaces around missing teeth.

• **Interdental picks** come in wood or plastic and many companies make them in various styles. I like ones called Stim-U-Dents®. They are wedge-shaped balsa wood sticks that, once softened in your mouth with your saliva, are flexible enough to be pushed in

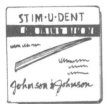

between your teeth, and poked in and out to almost "polish" the sides of the teeth. They are especially good to use while in the car, on the phone, or while watching TV. You don't have to look in the mirror; instead you can "feel" your way around. They come in a convenient package the size of a pack of matches.

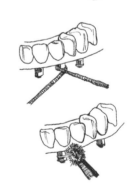

• **Yarn and pipe cleaners** are for those cavernous areas where a whole meal will stay for a week.

• **Implant loops** are an excellent way to remove bacteria around your implants without damaging the surrounding tissues. Since these are not too well known, ask your hygienist how to use them.

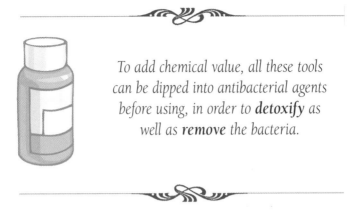

*To add chemical value, all these tools can be dipped into antibacterial agents before using, in order to **detoxify** as well as **remove** the bacteria.*

Tooth Whiteners

I would not suggest you start whitening your teeth during your pregnancy. While there are no studies that I know of that say they are unsafe, I always like to follow the adage "Better safe than sorry."

After your pregnancy, the only whiteners I would recommend are those from a reputable dentist. I am reluctant to recommend any over-the-counter whiteners that you buy in your local drug store or through TV offers.

On a personal note, I like to see someone with whiter teeth. It makes one look more youthful, more vital, and more confident, and is an added incentive to maintaining good oral hygiene.

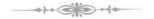

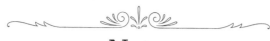

Notes

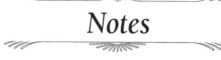

Chapter Eight

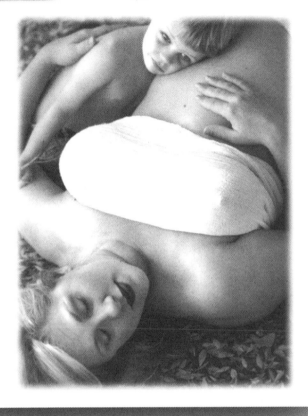

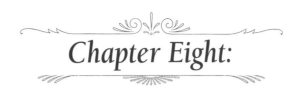

Chapter Eight:

Pregnancy and Whole Body Health

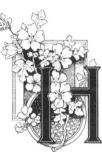ealth and wellness, in my opinion, are a natural result of balanced eating, balanced work and fun, balanced thinking, personal hygiene, spiritual nourishment, and positive attitudes about life. When one is happy and carefree, life looks wonderful. We experience youth independent of age, and vitality, excitement, self-expression, happiness, and wellness. When we are troubled, worried, laden down with heavy problems, we suffer uneasiness (dis-ease) in our physical body.

Is it any wonder that stress contributes to more than 50% of all illnesses?

In this chapter, I am going to talk with you about three things that I see as detrimental to your pregnancy, from the unique perspective of how they relate to your mouth: smoking, alcohol, and refined sugar. All three directly affect the tissues of the mouth and your potential for developing periodontal disease and dental decay during your pregnancy. I feel this last chapter is vital to round out the information you've learned so far.

The following information will help you make important personal decisions that affect not only you, but also your baby. And, when you pass them along to your child, they will positively influence your baby's babies, and your baby's babies' babies!

Thus the circle of life continues, and with it the handing down of knowledge that is so crucial to our continued development as mothers, as teachers, as individuals, as friends.

Let's start with smoking ... and other tobacco products.

Smoking

So many of the patients who have sat in my dental chair over the years were smokers. Some had smoked all their adult lives, and some were young people who had been smoking for only a few years. Regardless of the length of their addiction, their dangerous habits were affecting their mouths in much the same manner: Negatively!

Many of these patients have defensively told me, "I know you are going to tell me not to smoke." I always answer by saying, "I will let the facts speak for themselves." I do intend to tell you the facts, so you can make up your own mind about the risks of smoking during your pregnancy.

Cigarette smoking is widely reported as the single most preventable cause of premature death in the entire United States; 1 out of every 5 deaths in America is smoking-related. Tobacco use is linked with many serious illnesses such as cancer, lung disease, and heart disease, and numerous other health problems. Tobacco users also are at increased risk for gum infections; recent studies have shown that tobacco use may be one of the most significant risk factors in the development and progression of periodontal disease.

Certainly, if you do not presently smoke, I cannot imagine why you would ever want to start. Still, people young and old continue to do so, and at increasingly alarming rates. Each day, 6,000 young people will take their first puff on a cigarette. All told, half of that number will become — and stay — regular smokers. About two thirds of new smokers will eventually try to quit, yet few are successful — and close to 75% of them will still be smoking some seven to nine years after they lit their first cigarette.

In the United States, 23 % of all women and 27 % of reproductive-aged women smoke cigarettes. One study suggested that about 13 % of pregnant women in the United States smoke during pregnancy.

According to the U.S. Public Health Service, if all pregnant women in the U.S. stopped smoking, there would be an estimated 10 % reduction in infant deaths. A recent Danish study conducted over a six month period, reported that women who smoked were about 30 % less likely to conceive than non-smokers.

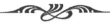

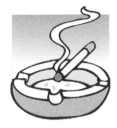 *Smokers are seven times more likely to develop periodontal infections than non-smokers. In one study, 40% of smokers lost their teeth by the end of their lives.*

It should come as no surprise to you that, where your mouth is concerned, the effects of smoking are direct — and significantly impact the sensitive tissues of your gums. This is mainly a result of the drying effect smoking has on your tongue, cheeks, gums, and palate. Nicotine is a *vasoconstrictor,* and reduces the supply of blood and nutrition to your tissues.

Because your mouth is generally a very moist place, thanks mainly to saliva and the fact that your mouth is closed for a considerable portion of the day, the heat and "drying out" effects caused by smoking create an environment that is entirely unnatural.

Bacteria that are normally washed away by saliva in a non-smoker's mouth tend to hang around and sit in places they're not wanted. Certain bacteria, the anaerobes, thrive in surroundings with reduced oxygen.

Several recent studies have provided evidence that tobacco smokers have poorer oral hygiene — and more dental tartar — perhaps due to a general lack of health consciousness.

Oral and pharyngeal cancers, those of the throat, windpipe, voice box, esophagus, and deep down into your lungs, can also develop more swiftly in the dry and irritated tissues of smokers.

Tobacco use greatly compromises our ability to fight off disease, so periodontal infections tend to get worse in the presence of cigarette smoke because the body's defense mechanisms are inhibited in smokers. Smoking also depletes Vitamin C, so necessary for healthy gum tissues. Some studies even suggest that smoking may accelerate bone loss.

Just a Pinch?

But those who smoke cigarettes are not the only folks at risk. What about their cigar and/or pipe-smoking brethren? *The Journal of the American Dental Association* reported in their January 1999 issue that both pipe and cigar smokers experienced bone and tooth loss as often as those who smoked the same amount of cigarettes.

And let's not forget those individuals who enjoy smokeless tobacco. Smokeless tobacco, often called "dip" or "chew" by its faithful fans, can also accelerate the risk of bone and fiber loss in and around the teeth, in addition to causing gum recession.

The effects can be even worse than that, however. One case in particular stands out in my mind: I once had a fourteen-year-old boy in my dental chair who "dipped" tobacco. He used to chew the tobacco and then hold it against his lower lip and gums when he played baseball because, he said, it was "cool."

When he came in to have his teeth cleaned, I noticed a suspicious-looking white patch between his cheek and gums, which had obviously developed from the constant irritation of a foreign, nicotine-soaked substance being placed there on a regular basis during baseball season. It definitely appeared to be pre-cancerous, and I told him that if he didn't stop "dipping," he would probably lose his jawbone — if not his very *life!*

He quit.

And lived ...

Please check out this web site for more information about smokeless tobacco: www.nstep.org.

According to the American Academy of Periodontology, as a smoker, or even as a user of non-smoking but tobacco-containing products, you are more likely than nonsmokers to have the following problems

- *Deep pockets between your teeth and gums.*

- *Loss of the bone and tissue that support your teeth.*

- *Calculus, plaque that hardens on your teeth that can only be removed during a professional cleaning.*

Enough said. The fact remains, however, that the choice is always yours. Whether you choose to use that extra butter to spread on your toast, to sit and watch one more TV show and forego your evening walk, to eat that chocolate bar, or to light up another cigarette, you are making choices that affect your overall body health every single day.

Some of them are good.

Some of them are not.

All of them affect the health of your mouth ...

Effects of Smoking on Pregnancy

But your teeth, mouth, and gums are not the only areas of your life to be affected by smoking. Smoking affects your pregnancy, and your unborn child, in the following negative ways:

- *Increases the risk of premature childbirth (before the 37th week) by about 30%.*

- *Increases the incidence of low-birth weight infants who weigh less than 5 1/2 pounds at birth.*

- *Increases the risk of stillbirths and deaths of babies in the first week of life by 33%.*

- *Stunts the growth and development of your baby.*

- *Increases pregnancy complications*

According to the July 1999 edition of *Oncology News International*, reporting on the findings of two studies presented at the annual meeting of the American Association for Cancer Research, "new research finds that even maternal exposure to second-hand smoke may harm the fetus." One of the studies, conducted by Steven R. Myers, Ph.D. and Dr. M.P. Ross of the University of Louisville School of Medicine, indicated that "exposure of expectant mothers to second-hand smoke is a major cause of concern because the unborn baby is also exposed to cancer-causing chemicals."

The Risk to Your Child

Just as smoking affects much more than just your mouth, yours is not the only life at risk as a result of cigarette smoke and other tobacco-containing products. What about your little one? Smoking puts the baby at increased risk for:

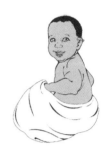

- *Genetic defects*

- *Sudden Infant Death Syndrome, or SIDS. Babies whose mothers smoke are twice as likely to die from SIDS. The risk is increased further if both parents smoke, compared to if only the mother smokes*

- *Stunted growth and development*

- *Miscarriage rates increase*

- *Asthma*

- *Respiratory infections*

- *Smoking increases the risk of premature labor. Premature labor is twice as common for smokers. It is an even bigger problem for women who smoke in the latter half of pregnancy*

- *Poor lung development*

- *Learning and behavioral problems. One study found that boys whose mothers smoked during pregnancy were four times more likely to have serious behavioral problems.*

The good news is that women who quit smoking before or during pregnancy reduce the risk for adverse reproductive outcomes. If a woman stops smoking by the 16th week of pregnancy, she's no more likely to have a low-birth weight baby than a woman who never smoked at all. In fact, eliminating maternal smoking might lead to a 10% reduction in all infant deaths.

Compelling Reasons to Quit

As if all this stuff isn't serious enough, Dr. Barry Solomon, author of *Keep Your Teeth in your Mouth for a Lifetime*, admonishes: "Smoking makes you look downright UGLY. Skin wrinkles add years of age to your appearance."

I thought you might like to hear a few encouraging reasons to quit smoking … if you are not already convinced.

- *If you smoke one pack of cigarettes a day, you will save over eighteen hundred dollars a year by quitting your habit. If you put only $1,000 (a bit more than half) of that money into the bank at 5% interest, in 20 years your baby would have $34,719.25 waiting for him or her!*

- *Nicotine and carbon monoxide start to leave your body within the first few hours after you quit smoking.*

- *Within 24 hours, your chance of a heart attack decreases significantly.*

- *Within two days of quitting smoking, your sense of taste and smell will improve.*

- *Most of the nicotine is gone from your body in 2-3 days, and your heart and lungs will immediately begin to repair the damage done by smoking.*

- *Within a month after stopping, blood pressure becomes normal.*

- *Three months after stopping, the lungs will have regained the capacity to clean themselves properly.*

- *Quitting smoking decreases the risk of many cancers, heart attack, stroke, and chronic lung disease. It can also increase life expectancy provided that quitting occurs before the onset of any major disease.*

There are many helpful and informative organizations eager to share more information with you about smoking. They include the American Cancer Society, the Mayo Clinic, and the American Heart Association. Any or all of these wonderful organizations can direct you to whatever additional resources you might need, including pamphlets, brochures, and other publications filled to the brim with facts and figures such as those listed above.

Alcohol

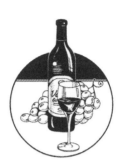

Found predominantly in wine, liquor, and beer, alcohol is another one of those items that should be eliminated altogether, or strictly limited, during pregnancy. Numerous studies have linked alcohol consumption with birth defects. It is a "drug" that really has no positive benefits, is high in calories, and offers nothing in the way of nutrition to the mother or forming fetus.

Furthermore, alcohol crosses into the placenta, transferring its toxicity to the baby's bloodstream. The more frequently one drinks, and the greater the quantity one consumes, the greater the risks of miscarriage, birth defects, retarded growth, and mental disorders in newborns.

A pregnant woman who drinks frequently and heavily is more likely to give birth to a child with a condition known as Fetal Alcohol Syndrome, the effects of which can even include malformations of the heart. Children with FAS can have problems with attention span, problem solving, learning, memory, speech, and even their hearing.

They can also have problems in school, as well as difficulties in socializing with other children. FAS is an irreversible, lifelong condition that affects every aspect of the child's life, as well as the lives of the child's family.

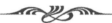

Important Note: There is no safe amount of alcohol that a woman can drink while she is pregnant. However, it is never too late to stop drinking. FAS is 100% preventable.

From studies done with over six thousand subjects, Dr. Sara Grossi at the University of Buffalo, New York, theorizes that alcohol use may increase the risk of periodontal infections in several ways, and the increase in risk is directly related to the quantity of alcohol consumed. We already know that periodontal infections increase one's risk for heart disease and other systemic problems, pregnancy consequences included. Alcohol and pregnancy don't mix. Enough said!

Refined Sugar

Refined sugar is not only bad for your teeth and gums, but it is also bad for your pregnancy. It provides only empty calories, adds weight, and can lead to diabetes, heart disease, and arthritis. We Americans eat entirely too much sugar — almost 7 tablespoons per person per day — which adds nothing in terms of nutrition to your daily need for nutrients, vitamins, and minerals.

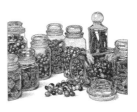

Sugar, in the presence of certain plaque-producing bacteria, leads to the production of bacterial byproducts that are very acidic in nature. These acids, if allowed to sit on the enamel of your teeth, cause demineralization of the tooth enamel and the underlying dentin. Eventually, this will cause a breakdown in the tooth structure and further bacterial invasion.

There are many factors that influence the development of dental caries. Here are some to consider:

- *The presence of plaque-producing bacteria (especially Strep Mutans and Lactobacilli)*

- *The susceptibility of tooth surfaces to decay (deep groves and fissures on biting surfaces, or margins around fillings)*

- *The frequency of eating and the types of snacks chosen (sugars and starches feed the bacteria)*

- *The quantity of saliva in the mouth (saliva neutralizes acid – a dry mouth makes one more prone to cavities)*

Sticky foods are more harmful than non-sticky foods because they stay in contact with the teeth longer. If you cannot brush immediately, I suggest taking a sip or two of water after eating things like raisins and pastries for example, to "swish and swallow" in order to wash away some of the foods that linger.

One other thing that is essential for you to know: When you *do* indulge in a sugary treat, it is better to eat candy or drink sweet liquids all in one sitting rather than to sip on a soda or take tiny bites of sweets all day long. Eating small bursts of sugar throughout your day is more damaging to your oral health because the bacteria are nourished for about 20 minutes each time you introduce sugar into your mouth.

I want you to remember that taking care of yourself is an ongoing process. You can't go back and erase all the fast food, packaged snacks, and junk you ate when you were a kid, last year, or even a week before you learned you were pregnant. However, you can make even the smallest changes today. Here's where we start:

Healthy Snack Alternatives

Here is a list of healthier alternatives to those quick, convenient, sugary snacks you often enjoyed before your pregnancy, but should reconsider now that you are thinking for two.

- *Yogurt with fresh fruit*

- *Fresh cheese*

- *Whole grain bagels, whole wheat toast, or bran muffins with cream cheese, peanut butter, or fruit spread*

- *Homemade frozen popsicles, using 1 6oz. can frozen concentrated juice mixed with a small container (6-8 oz.) of plain yogurt. I used to give these to my son when he was teething. They were yummy for both of us!*

- *Baked apples or other baked or stewed fruit*

- *Fresh fruit (Choose from a range of colors to insure variety of nutrients and vitamins)*

- *Fruit smoothies, homemade, using yogurt and banana as your base. Add other fruit and flavorings with ice to make a delicious drink*

- *Unsweetened whole grain cereal with yogurt and fresh fruit*

- *Nuts and seeds with natural dried fruit*

- *Celery with peanut butter (my personal favorite)*

- *Raw carrot sticks, cucumber slices, green pepper wedges (or any fresh vegetables, for that matter) with a dip made from yogurt, sour cream, or cottage cheese and herbs*

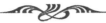

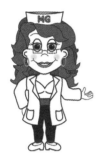
Mama Gums reminds you: Brush as quickly as possible after eating or drinking anything with a high sugar or starch content. By keeping these residues at a very low level, you reduce the nutrients many plaque-forming bacteria depend on for their growth and survival.

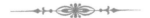

Notes

Afterword

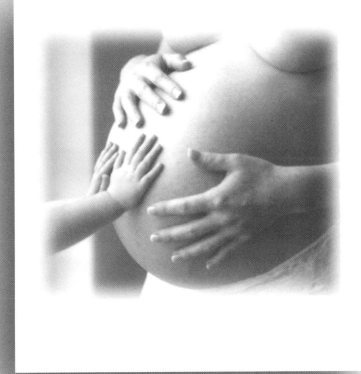

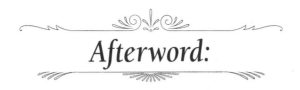

Afterword:

Here's to You and Your Baby

Well, that's it. I know I've said a "mouthful," but chances are you've learned some new ideas and concepts that will alter the way you have been doing things. Congratulations.

I hope you have enjoyed reading the book. I think it's important to relate the teeth, the gums, and the mouth with not only your pregnancy and your unborn child, but with your entire, overall body health as well. And I'm not alone. The Surgeon General's report substantiates the viewpoint that the mouth is the gateway to many illnesses. Keeping your mouth healthy is a step on the path towards a long, healthy life.

As you now know, it's important to arm yourself with all of the most relevant facts currently available — and to then act accordingly. Most of the information I've offered is preventative, and it is my sincere hope that you and your baby have long lives with healthy teeth and gums. Being pregnant is a miraculous, joyous experience, and I wish you good health and happiness with your new arrival.

If at any time before, during, or after your pregnancy you should ever have any questions or comments, please come visit me at my web site, www.mamagums.com. There you will find the latest information on teeth, gums, and total body concerns, and other useful resources as well. Also, you can always e-mail me at Mamagums@aol.com not just with questions, comments, or concerns, but with news about your newborn child!

I wish you nothing but the most flawless and effortless pregnancy ever, and a safe and healthy delivery to look back on for many years to come. The birth of your child is not just the end of your pregnancy, but the beginning of a marvelous relationship that will last a lifetime.

You have already proven yourself to be an avid collector of information. After all, how many pregnant women eagerly seek out information about their mouths when it's their bellies that are getting all the attention? This inherent hunger for knowledge will stand you in good stead as you and your child enjoy your lives together.

Thanks for spending this very special time with me. We are just about finished. I have included a Tour of the Mouth in Appendix I, which I consider optional but interesting reading. Also included in Appendix II is important information about vitamins and supplements. This information was contributed by a wonderful holistic dentist named Dr. Tom Baldwin. Dr. Baldwin's dental practice is located at 7801 York Road in Towson, Maryland. Phone: (410) 321-0558. His web site is: http://nontoxicdentistry.com. His impressive credentials include: DDS., MAGD, (Mastership in the Academy of General Dentistry), F/AIAOMT, (Fellow Accredited in the International Academy of Oral and Medical Toxicology), BS in Psychology, Masters in Holistic Nutrition, Clayton College of Natural Health, in process.

Just one more thing. Now that you are nearly through with the book, why not take a break, put your feet up, and enjoy some quiet time all to yourself. Choose a place where you know you won't be disturbed and give yourself at least 30 minutes to meditate or breathe deeply. Perhaps you'll light a few candles and surround yourself with a beautiful fragrance or lovely fresh flowers. Let the feelings of warmth, peacefulness and calm wash over you and try to keep that feeling of serenity with you for the rest of the day.

Ahhhhhhhhhhh.

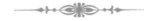

Appendices

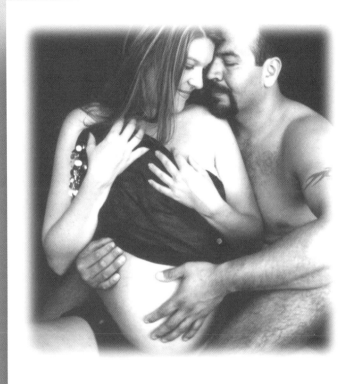

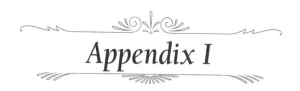

Appendix I

Tour of the Mouth

When we think of our mouths, we usually go no further than what we can see on the outside, our lips. However, the lips are only the outermost threshold of a complex and amazing cavity that is home to some of the human body's most fascinating structures.

Have you ever really peeked *inside* your mouth? Really gone in deep for a closer look at the magical portal through which every morsel of food you've ever eaten has passed? Ever peered farther than the bristles of your toothbrush might go? Ever stuck out your tongue and marveled at the thousands of nooks and crannies on its limitless surface?

What's that you say?

Not lately?

Well, you're not alone. Most people never really look into their mouths unless there is something wrong. Sore throat? Swollen glands? Something stuck between the teeth? But to the entire dental profession, as it might soon be to you, the mouth is a fascinating place full of deep, dark caverns, glistening, moist walls, dangling stalactites, and other amazing features. Let's have some fun …

What do you say?

Go get a mirror and a good, strong light …

Now, open wide … let's Take a Tour of the Mouth!

There are many stops on our *Tour of the Mouth*. Some spots may be prettier than others; some spots might be downright unsightly, but I can guarantee you this: you won't get bored along the way!

You'll learn things you never knew. You may even re-learn about some things you might have forgotten from sixth grade biology.

Anatomical Tour of the Mouth

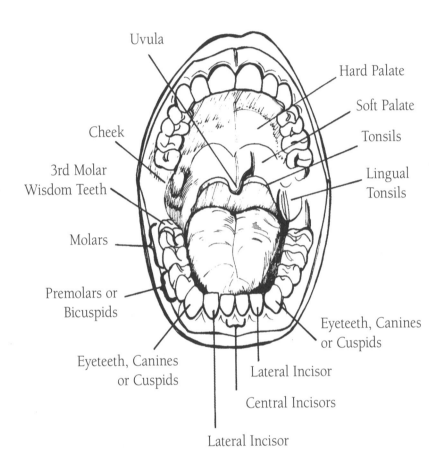

Uvula

Hard Palate

Soft Palate

Tonsils

Cheek

Lingual
Tonsils

3rd Molar
Wisdom Teeth

Molars

Premolars or
Bicuspids

Eyeteeth, Canines
or Cuspids

Eyeteeth, Canines
or Cuspids

Lateral Incisor

Central Incisors

Lateral Incisor

The main things you'll see along our Tour of the Mouth are:

- The Tongue
- The Cheeks
- The Palates, hard and soft
- The Tonsils
- The Uvula
- The Teeth

The Tongue

The tongue is not only the principal organ of taste, it is also vital to speech, aids in chewing and swallowing, and even has untold uses in the field of human communication. For instance, as an expression of dislike or disdain for someone, to stick out the tongue is an extremely effective, if childish, gesture!

The surface of the tongue contains three different types of taste buds. The different taste sensations of sweet, salty, sour, and bitter are not only stimulating to your taste buds — but to the rest of your mouth as well. To better help you visualize just where exactly those taste buds "live" on your tongue, I have provided the following diagram:

Taste Buds

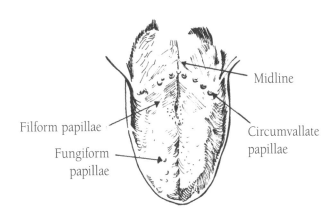

Midline

Filform papillae

Circumvallate papillae

Fungiform papillae

Taste buds, clearly evident at birth, are found on the tip, back, and sides of the tongue. Like tennis shoes or brake pads, the taste buds at the tip of your sensitive tongue tend to "wear out" and must be replaced every two weeks or so. The number of taste buds diminishes as we get older, but take heart. According to the Surgeon General's report, there appears to be "considerable reserve capacity, so there is normally little loss in the sense of taste as we age."

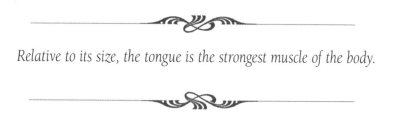

Relative to its size, the tongue is the strongest muscle of the body.

The Cheeks

The soft, fatty cushions on the sides of our mouths are called the cheeks — otherwise known as the exact spot your great aunt Millie is most likely to kiss you on in front of all of your friends!

This skin inside them, like all of the skin covering parts of our insides that open to the outside, is covered with mucous membranes. These vital mucous membranes are a specialized skin covering that lubricates and protects sensitive tissues from drying out.

The cheek muscles are very loose and carry the salivary ducts of the parotid glands, from which the saliva enters the mouth. There are also two other sets of salivary glands located under the tongue and under the floor of the mouth.

Although they are shaved, blushed, powdered, rouged, and occasionally even pinched on a daily basis, it is amazing to think how little we really know about the cheeks. As an example, here is a story to illustrate how little most people know about their own mouths.

One day a patient came in to see me, thoroughly convinced that he had cancer of the mouth. When I asked him why he had made this scary self-diagnosis, he said that he had just noticed "this thing on the inside of my cheek" and was convinced that it must be nothing short of a malignant growth. As I palpated the area in question, right around his upper molar, I asked him if this was the "growth" he had felt. He said yes, and I immediately showed him the same raised area on the *other* cheek. I then explained that these are called the Stenson's ducts through which the saliva flows into his mouth.

Needless to say, he was very relieved.

The Palates
(Hard & Soft)

The "hard palate" is a structure of bone that forms the front two thirds of the roof of the mouth. The back third, covered by muscles and tendons, is called the "soft palate." This soft tissue separates the nose from the mouth and allows food to go down into the esophagus without passing into the nasal cavity.

An occasional glitch when the bones of the hard palate don't close at birth is called a *cleft palate*, and people who have this condition either have surgery to protect it or wear an appliance called an "obturator" to make it easier to both eat and speak.

The palate is often the location for *palatine Tori*, benign bony projections or overgrowths of bone that make it difficult for some people to wear dentures. (All the more reason to keep your natural teeth for your lifetime.)

The Tonsils

The tonsils are actually bundles of lymph tissues covered with mucous membranes that are located in the mouth and down the throat. When we talk about "having our tonsils removed," we are actually talking about only one out of the three sets of tonsils that we possess. In fact, we are referring to the tonsils that are positioned at the far end of our mouths, the *palatine tonsils*, which guard the entrance to the tubes that extend to the lungs and digestive system. If you have ever experienced something "go down the wrong pipe," then you immediately know what I'm talking about!

The *pharyngeal tonsils*, when enlarged, are called *adenoids* and occasionally cause middle ear problems. Very little of these two types of tonsils is visible to you. The third type of tonsils, known as the *lingual tonsils*, are located on the sides of the tongue. The function of these tonsils is to act as a small filtration system to the lymphatic vessels and paranasal sinuses.

The Uvula

Despite its mysterious name, the uvula is actually one of the most recognizable features of the mouth — that little dangly piece of flesh at the rear of the soft palate! The uvula varies greatly in size and shape from person to person. Still, anomalies occur. In thirty years I have seen two people who were born with no uvula, and one who had a double uvula, called a "bifurcated uvula."

The uvula is formed during development in infancy, as the palate joins up from front to back. It works with the soft palate to seal off the nasal cavity during swallowing, regurgitation, and speaking. It may also play a minor role in clearing saliva from the oral cavity. If you're curious, many animals have uvulas, too!

The Teeth

As our *Tour of the Mouth* continues, we've enjoyed a quick refresher course on the Cheek, The Tongue, and even The Tonsils. But what would our tour be without stopping to check out those chompers for which the mouth is so famous?

In our discussion of the teeth, we will run across the following items: the crown, the neck, the root, the enamel, cementum, dentin, the pulp and pulp cavity, the root canal, the periodontal ligament, the alveolar socket, the gingiva, the canines, and the premolars. (Phew! Okay, now, say *that* three times fast! But be careful not to get your uvula in a knot!)

Don't be alarmed by their big, or perhaps even unfamiliar-sounding names. By the time our tour is over, you'll be able to impress both your friends and family with what you've learned on your *Tour of the Mouth*.

The Crown

The crown, or "clinical crown," is generally the part of the tooth extending above the gum line. It can occasionally get longer with recession of the gums, or perhaps due to gum disease or even surgery. There is currently some disagreement as to whether recession is a part of the natural aging process. The "anatomical crown" is that part of the tooth covered with enamel, which can get smaller over time due to erosion, abrasion, or *bruxism*, more commonly known as "tooth grinding."

The Neck

The neck of the tooth is where the crown meets the root. The technical name is the Cemento-Enamel Junction, or "CEJ."

The Root

That part of the tooth that extends into the jawbone is known as the root. Incisors and canine teeth have a single root. Molars have one, two (bifurcated), or three (trifurcated) roots, depending on their type and location in the mouth.

Parts of a Tooth

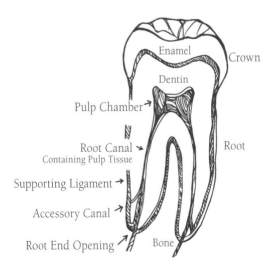

Enamel

Enamel is the protective material that covers the crown of the tooth. Although it is the hardest living substance in the body, enamel is very brittle and prone to cracking and chipping. One favorite summer pastime, chewing on ice cubes, is a culprit in cracking enamel, and should naturally be avoided. Other damage to the crown's enamel, such as staining, can result from coffee, tea, smoking, and poor oral hygiene. However, unlike cracking, a dentist or hygienist can often remove these unsightly stains with polishing.

Cementum

Cementum is the material that covers the roots of the teeth. Not as hard as enamel, cementum nonetheless attaches itself to fibers that help anchor the tooth to the jawbone and its integrity is thus vital to good oral health.

Dentin

Dentin is a bone-like substance found underneath the enamel and cementum that makes up most of the tooth structure, and actually gives the tooth its color.

The Pulp and Pulp Cavity

In the center of the tooth, a "living" area known as the pulp cavity, contains the blood vessels, nerves, and connective tissue that together comprise the pulp. It is vital to the overall health of your mouth, because its blood supply provides nutrients that help keep the tooth alive.

The Pulp Canal or Root Canal

The pulp or root canal is the space through which blood vessels and nerves enter the tooth. When a tooth "dies," or becomes non-vital, some dentists believe it is time for a root canal procedure in order to avoid extraction. This involves removing the dead nerve, sterilizing the canal, and filling it with a rubber-like material called *gutta-percha*. There are other less commonly known materials like calcium oxide root fillings and thermoplastic materials. The local anesthetics used in modern dentistry make discomfort from root canals a thing of the past.

There are some strong opinions against root canal therapy presented by Dr. Westin Price, a respected researcher who studied the potential serious side effects of the procedure for over 25 years. His scientific data suggests that root canal therapy is the cause of many systemic diseases and illnesses. He suggests that the health of a person's immune system must be considered, and if a person has chronic health problems, existing root canal filled teeth or untreated dead teeth should be considered as a possible cause or influence. For more information, please contact the **International Academy of Oral and Medical Toxicology** at: www.iaomt.org or in Florida, at: Tel: (863) 420-6373. You will also find interesting information about the mercury toxicity of amalgam fillings and the controversy surrounding fluoridation, as well as a list of wonderful doctors and dentists who truly care about holistic healing.

The Periodontal Ligament

The periodontal ligament contains bundles of tissue fibers that connect the cementum to the alveolar, or bone, socket and anchors the teeth within the jawbone.

The Alveolar Process and Socket

The alveolar socket is the crater-like opening in the jawbone that actually holds the tooth. Its walls are called "the alveolar process," and develop around the teeth when they first emerge through the gums.

The Gingiva

The gingiva is the pink flesh that covers the jawbone and fits snugly around the neck of the tooth. When covered in a more callused tissue called keratin, the gums are thus thicker and more resistant to the injuries that result from the normal wear and tear that the mouth endures every day. When we eat hot pizza, chew hard, crunchy foods, poke ourselves with a sharp object, or are exposed to bacteria, our gum tissues, when intact, protect us from any intruders.

The Types of Teeth

Animals' teeth reflect their diets. For instance, meat eaters like lions, wolves, and dogs, have sharp, pointed teeth with which to pierce and tear their prey. Plant eaters like horses and cows, on the other hand, have broad, flat teeth with which to crush and grind. Humans, with our varied diet of both soft and hard foods consisting of both plants and animals, have different types of teeth in order to handle both types of food.

These types of human teeth include the incisors, the canines, the premolars, and the molars.

Types of Permanent Teeth

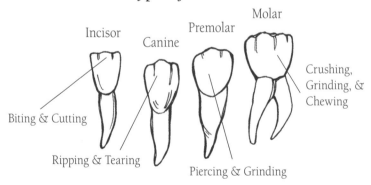

Incisor — Biting & Cutting

Canine — Ripping & Tearing

Premolar — Piercing & Grinding

Molar — Crushing, Grinding, & Chewing

The Incisors

The four front teeth in the upper and lower jaws are known as the incisors. The central pairs of these instantly recognizable teeth are understandably called the "central incisors." The teeth on either side of the central incisors are known as the lateral incisors. Incisors are broad, flat teeth with a narrow cutting edge and a single root, designed for biting and cutting.

The Canines

The four teeth on both sides of your upper and lower incisors are known as the canines, although they are sometimes referred to as the eyeteeth or cuspids. Canines come to a single sharp point for ripping and tearing at tough foods, and for piercing and holding. They also have a single root.

The Premolars

There are a total of eight premolars, or bicuspids. These complex and useful teeth combine points for piercing with broader surfaces for grinding. The upper first premolars, located next to the canines, have two roots, while the second premolars have but one. All lower premolars have one root.

The Molars

Molars are the last three teeth on both sides of your mouth, both in the upper and lower jaws. The first molars appear in the mouth at around age 6, the second molars at age 12 and the third molars, also called wisdom teeth, appear between 17 and 21. Not everyone gets wisdom teeth. They are frequently missing or sometimes impacted. Molars are very specialized teeth that have broad surfaces for crushing, grinding, and chewing. Upper molars have three roots, while the lower molars have but two.

Numbering Systems

At the often busy and even more precise dentist's office, describing a problem tooth with words to the effect of "the big one toward the back on the left," just doesn't cut it! With typically thirty-two teeth in the human mouth, standardized systems of numbering and identification are absolutely necessary in order to identify individual teeth quickly and efficiently.

Understanding the numbering systems currently used in dental offices all over the country will help you to better understand what your dentist is actually *doing* in your mouth. The two most common systems are the Universal Numbering System and the Palmer Notation Method, the former being used by the ADA and most general dentists, the latter in use by many oral surgeons and orthodontists.

In the Universal Numbering System, the back molar on your upper right side is considered "Number 1." To remain standard, both removed and missing teeth are still counted. In other words, if you've had your wisdom teeth removed and "Number 1" is actually missing in action, your dentist will start with "Number 2" instead.

Numbering goes right to left across the front to the farthest back on the upper left side, which is "Number 16." The farthest tooth back on the lower left is "Number 17," and from there back across to the lower right back for "Number 32."

In the Palmer Notation Method, the mouth is divided into four "quadrants." Numbering is the same for each quadrant, from 1 at the center of the mouth to 8 at the back, with unique symbols differentiating the quadrants. In other words, 8 teeth in each quadrant (4) still equals 32 (8 x 4) teeth.

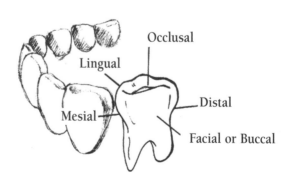

Five Tooth Surfaces

Other jargon that you need to know in order to be a "savvy consumer" at the dentist's office refers to the sides, or "surfaces," of the individual teeth. The "buccal" surface is the outside of the tooth, or the side facing your cheek or lips. In the front of the mouth it is sometimes called the facial or labial surface.

The "lingual" surface is the inside of the tooth, or the side toward your tongue. On upper teeth this is sometimes called the palatal surface. The sides between the teeth are the "mesial" (facing the center) and "distal" (facing the rear). The top surface of a tooth is known as the "occlusal." Raised parts of the occlusal are called "cusps," while indented parts are called "grooves."

The End of Our Tour!

Well, that's it! I hope you've enjoyed the guided tour through the mysterious mouth. You are now amongst the select minority who can decifer the gibberish you hear in your dentist's office. Bravo and congratulations!

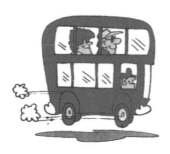

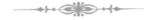

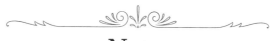

Notes

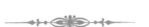

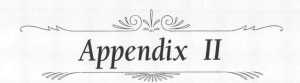

Appendix II

Dr. Thomas Baldwin's Pregnancy Protocol

Vitamins

- **Vitamin A**   2000-3,000 mg
- **B-Complex**   50 mg
- **Folic Acid**   800mcg
- **Vitamin C**   2,000 mg
- **Vitamin E**   100 IU's
- **Vitamin D**   400 IU's
- **Calcium Citrate**   800 mg
- **Magnesium**   600 mg
- **Zinc**   25 mg
- **Iodine**   150-300 mcg and/or through diet (seafood, salt)
- **Carnitine**   500-1,000 mg
- **Fish Oil**   3 grams per day
- **Copper**   2-4 mg

If you have nausea, Vitamin B6 is useful in doses of 25-50 mg per day and has been found to be safe and effective.

Foods that are really great for you to eat are:

- Fish (but not mackerel, swordfish, or tuna ... due to mercury)

- Shellfish

- Salmon (Like all fish, it is important where it comes from. The Great Northwest is good. Pen-raised is bad. If you cannot determine where it comes from, avoid it!)

- Meat and dairy (preferably organic)

- Butter (never margarine!)

- Extra Virgin olive oil

- Coconut oil (for cooking)

- Plenty of fresh vegetables

- Whey protein

- Bee pollen

- Nutritional yeast

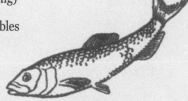

Eggs are also very important for you to eat (especially free-range organic eggs). Eggs are almost a perfect food, and are not bad for either a Type I or Type II diet!!! A couple of eggs a day would be excellent.

Good Practice:

- Limit alcohol severely
- Do not take any herbs without consulting your OB or me!

Things to Avoid:

- Trans fatty acids
- Processed foods
- Commercial baked goods
- Margarine
- Movie popcorn
- All vegetable shortening
- All partially hydrogenated oils

The reason Coconut oil is better for baking is that it is not damaged by heat. It is almost 50% lauric acid (found in high quantities in breast milk) which is a powerful anti-microbial substance, and most of the remaining saturates are in the short and medium chain form, which are used for energy and not stored as body fat.

If You Have Gestational Diabetes:

- Chromium in doses of 200-400 mcg per day has been found to be safe and effective.
- Zinc and magnesium are also important to optimize.

Fats and cholesterol are very important to growing babies, both in utero and for the first years of life. That's why the fish oil is so important.

Breast-feeding:

When the baby is born, if you choose to breast-feed (I recommend that highly) and you find that milk production is insufficient, sage and fennel can be used safely to promote better milk production through raising prolactin levels. 1-3 cups of each as a tea or 1-3 droppers of each as a tincture may be used daily. Adjust dose as breast milk production changes.

Dr. Thomas Baldwin

A Special Precaution from Mama Gums: It is never advisable to have any x-rays, including dental x-rays, taken during the first three months of your pregnancy. That is a critical time in the development of your baby. It is preferable to wait until your baby is born before having any x-rays unless you have a dental emergency, and then a protective lead shield should be used. A few dentists are now using digital x-rays, which have the potential to reduce exposure significantly while sacrificing only slightly in the quality of the picture.

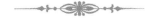

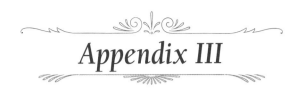

Appendix III

Helpful Organizations and Web sites

- **American Academy of Periodontology**

  737 N. Michigan Avenue, Suite 800
  Chicago, IL 60611-2690
  Phone: 312-787-5518
  Fax: 312-787-3670
  Web site: www.perio.org

- **American Red Cross National Headquarters**

  431 18th Street, NW
  Washington, DC 20006
  Phone: 202-303-4498
  Web site: www.redcross.org

- **Healthfinder**

  (Web site of the Department of Health and Human Services)
  P.O. Box 1133
  Washington, DC 20013-1133
  E-mail: healthfinder@nhic.org
  Web site: www.healthfinder.gov

- **La Leche League International**

  P.O. Box 4079
  Schaumburg, IL 60168-4079
  Phone: 847-519-7730
  Toll-free 800-LALECHE
  Fax: 847-519-0035
  Order Department: 847-519-9585
  Web Site: www.lalecheleague.org

- **Lamaze International**

  2025 M Street
  Suite 800
  Washington, DC 20036-3309
  Local: 202-367-1128
  Toll-free: 800-368-4404
  Fax: 202-367-2128
  Web Site: www.lamaze.org

- **March of Dimes**

  1275 Mamaroneck Avenue
  White Plains, NY 10605
  Web Site: www.marchofdimes.com

- **The National Women's Health Information Center**

  A project of the US Department of Health and Human Services, Office of Women's Health
  8550 Arlington Boulevard, Suite 300
  Fairfax, VA 22031
  1-800-994 WOMAN or 1-888-220-5446 for the hearing impaired
  Phone lines open Monday – Friday, 9 am to 6 pm EST
  Web sites: www.4woman.gov

- **Office of the Surgeon General**

  5600 Fishers Lane
  Room 18-66
  Rockville, MD 20857
  Web site: www.surgeongeneral.gov

- **The Office on Women's Health**

  Department of Health and Human Services
  200 Independence Avenue, SW Room 730B
  Washington, DC 20201
  Phone: 202-690-7650
  Fax: 202-205-2631

- **Smoke Free Families**

  National Program Office:
  University of Alabama at Birmingham
  1530 3rd Avenue S
  Birmingham, AL 35294-1150
  Phone: 205-934-4011
  National Dissemination Office: University of North Carolina at Chapel Hill
  E-Mail: info@smokefreefamilies.org
  Web Site: www.smokefreefamilies.org

- **United States Department of Health and Human Services**

  National Institutes of Health
  9000 Rockville Pike
  Bethesda, MD 20892
  Phone: 301-496-4000
  Phone lines open Monday – Friday, 9 am to 4 pm Eastern Time
  Web Site: www.nih.gov/health/infoline.htm

- **United States National Library of Medicine**

  8600 Rockville Pike
  Bethesda, MD 20894
  Web Site: www.nlm.nih.gov/medlineplus/mplusdictionary.html

For information regarding doctors/dentists who practice biological dentistry, contact the following organizations:

- **International Academy of Oral and Medical Toxicology (IAOMT)**

  8297 ChampionsGate Boulevard Suite #193
  ChampionsGate, FL 33896
  Phone: 863-420-6373
  Fax: 863-420-6394
  E-mail: info@iaomt.org
  Web Site: www.iaomt.org
  Dr. Michael Ziff....407-298-2450

- **International Dental Health Alliance**

  800-368-3396

- **Holistic Dental Association**

  P.O. Box 5007
  Durango, CA 81301
  Dr. Richard Shepard

- **The Academy of Biological Dentistry**

  408-659-5385

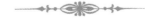

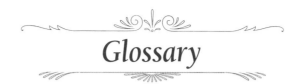

Glossary

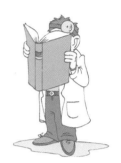

- **Abscess:** Localized collection of pus in a cavity formed by the breakdown of tissue cells.

- **Acute condition:** is a type of illness or injury that has a rapid onset and ordinarily lasts less than 3 months. (Pregnancy is also considered to be an "acute condition" despite lasting longer than 3 months).

- **Anaerobic bacteria:** Those organisms that cannot live in the presence of oxygen.

- **Antibiotics:** These drugs are used to combat both minor and life-threatening bacterial infections.

- **Bicuspids:** Also called premolars, are the two teeth behind the cuspids or eyeteeth. There are a total of 8.

- **Birth weight:** According to the National Center for Health Statistics, is defined as the first weight of the newborn obtained after birth.

  Low birth weight is defined as less than 2,500 grams or 5 pounds 8 ounces.

  Very low birth weight is defined as less than 1,500 grams or 3 pounds 4 ounces.

- **Calculus:** Hard, calcified dental plaque. It is the mineralized remains of dead bacteria attached to surfaces of the teeth. Also called "tartar." There are two types of calculus: that which forms above the gingival margins, called supragingival calculus, and that which forms on roots below the gingival margins, called subgingival calculus.

- **Canine or Cuspids:** Eyeteeth.

- **Caries or Dental Caries:** Tooth decay.

- **Carious lesion:** An area of decay on a tooth.

- **Cavitron:** Ultrasonic dental tool that uses high frequency sound waves to remove hard deposits from the teeth.

- **Cementum:** Hard tissue that covers the roots of teeth. Teeth are held in place by connective tissue fibers, the periodontal ligament that attaches the cementum to the bony sockets in the jaws.

- **Charting:** To record the depth of the gum pockets around teeth.

- **Chlorhexidine:** An anti-microbial agent effective in controlling gum diseases.

- **Debridement:** Removal of infection from a wound.

- **Dental caries:** Tooth decay

- **Dentifrice:** Any preparation used in the cleaning of the teeth.

- **Dentin:** Hard, living inner layer of a tooth just below the enamel layer.

- **Distal:** The surface that faces toward the back, away from the midline of the jaw.

- **Dry mouth:** (xerostomia) This occurs when the salivary glands in your mouth don't produce enough moisture, disrupting the balance of normal microorganisms in your mouth. This dryness increases your risk of oral thrush (yeast), dental caries, and periodontal infections.

- **Enamel:** The hardest substance of the body, the covering of the crown of the tooth, located above the gum line.

- **Eye teeth:** The four canines or cuspids.

- **Facial:** Pertaining to the face. The outer side of a tooth, that side facing the face.

- **Flap surgery:** Loosening of gums from bone to expose and debride the periodontal pocket as well as the underlying tooth structures.

- **Gestational Diabetes:** Approximately 3 percent to 5 percent of pregnant women in the United States develop gestational diabetes, a type of diabetes mellitus, usually beginning in the second or third trimester of pregnancy. Like other forms of diabetes, it affects the way your body uses blood sugar (glucose). In many cases it goes away after pregnancy, but more than 50% of women who experience this condition later develop a permanent form of diabetes - type 2 (formerly called adult-onset or noninsulin-dependent) diabetes.

- **Gingiva, gingivae:** The anatomical word for the gums.

- **Gingival:** The adjective pertaining to the gums.

- **Gingivectomy:** Surgery to remove gum tissue.

- **Gingivitis:** The initial stage of gum disease that is caused by pathogenic bacteria that reside in the gingival crevices (under the gums.) This initial stage of gingival disease may progress into destructive periodontitis. The gums usually become red, swollen, bleed easily, and are often tender to touch.

- **Incisors:** Four upper and four lower front teeth, the central and lateral incisors (excludes the canine teeth).

- **Implant:** Artificial device usually made from titanium, surgically placed in the jaw to substitute for a natural tooth root. Prosthetic teeth and bridges are attached to the part of the implant that protrudes through the gum. An implant functions like a natural tooth and needs to have the same care or will be lost through the same process of infection, called peri-implantitis rather than periodontitis.

- **Lavage:** Washing out or cleansing with water.

- **Lingual:** Pertaining to the tongue. That side of a tooth that faces the tongue.

- **Maintenance or recall therapy:** An ongoing program, designed to supplement the anti-infective self-care that patients use at home. This treatment, usually every 3-4 months, includes the professional examination of teeth and periodontal tissues for evidence of disease activity. Teeth are then scaled and polished, and pockets are irrigated with an antiseptic solution.

- **Malocclusion:** "Bad bite" between the upper and lower teeth, causing your teeth to align incorrectly.

- **Mandible:** The lower jaw.

- **Maxilla:** The upper jaw.

- **Mesial:** The surface (of the tooth) that faces closer to the front or to the midline of the jaw.

- **Microbiological:** Pertaining to microorganisms and their effects on other living organisms.

- **Molars:** The three back teeth in each quarter of the mouth, including the wisdom teeth.

- **Morning sickness:** The overall queasiness, nausea, or vomiting that many pregnant women experience during the first 12 to 14 weeks of their pregnancy.

- **Occlusal:** The surface of the tooth that is used for chewing.

- **Occlusion:** How the upper and lower teeth come together.

- **Oral hygiene:** The process of maintaining the cleanliness of the mouth.

- **Osseointegration:** The attachment and assimilation of the bone to a dental implant. This process takes from three to six months after the implant has been placed in the mouth.

- **Palatine, Palatal:** Related to the hard or soft palate.

- **Papilla, Papillae:** The cone shaped portion of gum tissue between the teeth.

- **Partial:** Removable denture replacing some of the teeth often lost through gum disease.

- **Pathogenic:** Disease-causing.

- **Peridex®:** Chlorhexidine.

- **Periodontal ligament:** The fibers of tissue that attach the teeth to the bone. When these ligaments are destroyed by advanced cases of periodontal disease, the teeth become loose.

- **Periodontal pocket:** A separation of the gum tissues surrounding the tooth forming a space or pocket. The pocket fills with plaque and infection. If not treated, the bone and connective tissue surrounding the tooth may become so severely damaged that the tooth will fall out or need to be extracted.

- **Periodontal disease(s):** Include gingivitis, rapidly advancing destructive periodontitis, and chronic destructive periodontitis.

- **Periodontitis, Periodontal disease, Periodontal infections, Destructive Periodontitis:** Infections caused by invasive bacteria that colonize root surfaces and the periodontal tissues that surround them.

Various types of periodontal disease affect about 80% of the American adult population. Untreated, destructive periodontitis will progress until the body, trying to protect itself, will cause the teeth to loosen and eventually fall out.

- **Periodontium:** The tissues that surround and support the teeth, including the gums, periodontal ligament and bone.

- **Periodontopathic:** Causing periodontal diseases.

- **Permanent teeth:** The thirty-two adult teeth.

- **Plaque or dental plaque:** Also called bacterial biofilms. These soft, sticky coatings form as many strains of bacteria colonize and grow on tooth surfaces above and below the gum margins. If plaque is not removed carefully each day by brushing, irrigating, and flossing, bacteria attached to tooth-surfaces die and harden from the minerals in the saliva and crevicular exudates. These mineralized deposits are called calculus or tartar.

- **Pregnancy:** An extraordinary chain of events that begins with the union of egg and sperm and the preparation of the body to provide the nourishment and hormones that govern the baby's growth and development.

- **Pregnancy Tumor:** A large lump or overgrowth of gum tissue that is not cancerous, generally is not painful, and usually disappears or diminishes after pregnancy. If the tumor persists, it may require removal by a periodontist or oral surgeon.

- **Proximal:** The surfaces nearest to or next to.

- **Pyogenic Granuloma:** Another name for pregnancy tumor.

- **Root:** The below the gum part of the tooth that anchors the tooth to the bone.

- **Root scaling and planing:** A non-surgical procedure where the hygienist, dentist, or periodontist removes soft bacterial plaques and their calcified remains (calculus) from tooth surfaces and periodontal pockets.

- **Sloughing:** (as related to the mouth) the casting off of the outside layer of skin or gum tissue.

- **Specific Plaque Hypothesis:** asserts that *specific* bacteria cause gum infections. The culprits are: Porphyromonas gingivalis, Bacteroides forsythus, and Treponema denticola.

- **Sub gingival:** Below the gum line.

- **Supra gingival:** Above the gum line.

- **Tartar:** A synonym for calculus.

- **Tempromandibular Joint:** (TMJ) the joint that links the two jaws, the maxilla and the mandible.

- **Therasol®:** A pleasant tasting, non-staining, anti-infective medication that can be used as a rinse or, when mixed with water, as an irrigating solution.

- **Tori:** Plural for torus.

- **Torus:** A benign outgrowth of bone that usually develops on the roof of the mouth or under the tongue, on the lower jawbone.

- **Uvula:** The little dangling structure in the back of your throat.

- **Vasoconstrictor:** Something that causes the narrowing of blood vessels so that less blood is able to flow through at a time.

- **Xerostomia:** See "dry mouth."

- **Xylitol chewing gum:** (pronounced zy-li-tall) A gum containing a natural sweetener made from the bark of birch trees. Recent studies show that xylitol gum helps to reduce the levels of Streptococcus Mutans, the bacteria responsible for dental caries.

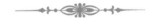

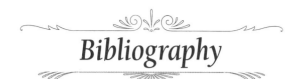

Bibliography

Armitage GC. Periodontal diseases: diagnosis. Ann Periodontol 1996;1:37-215.

Cali, Vincent M. *The New, Lower Cost Way to End Gum Trouble Without Surgery*. New York, N.Y.: Warner Books, Inc. 1982

Centers for Disease Control (CDC). Cigarette smoking among adults—United States, 1988. JAMA 1991 Dec 11;266(22):3113-4.

Centers for Disease Control (CDC). Preventing tobacco use among young people: a report of the Surgeon General. Executive summary. MMWR Morb Mortal Wkly Rep 1994b Mar 11;(RR-4):1-10.

Febres C, Echeverri EA, Keene HJ. Parental awareness, habits, and social factors and their relationship to baby bottle tooth decay. Pediatr Dent 1997 Jan-Feb;19(1):22-7.

Fiske J, Davis DM, Frances C, Gelbier S. The emotional effects of tooth loss in edentulous people. Brit Dent J 1998;184(2):90-3.

Genco RJ. Current view of risk factors for periodontal diseases. J Periodontol 1996 Oct;67(10 Suppl):1041-9.

Genco RJ. Risk factors for periodontal disease. In: Rose LF, Genco RJ, Cohen DW, Mealey BL, editors. Periodontal medicine. Hamilton (Ontario): B.C. Decker Inc.; 2000.

Gibbs RS, Romero R, Hillier SL, Eschenbach DA, Sweet RL. A review of premature birth and subclinical infection. Am J Obstet Gynecol 1992 May;166(5):1515-28.

Grossi SG, Skrepcinski FB, DeCaro T, Zambon JJ, Cummins D, Genco RJ. Response to periodontal therapy in diabetics and smokers. J Periodontol 1996 Oct;67(10 Suppl):1094-102.

Herzberg MC, MacFarlane GD, Liu P, Erickson PR. The platelet as an inflammatory cell in periodontal diseases: interactions with Porphyromonas gingivalis. In: Genco R, Hamada S, Lehner T, McGhee J, Mergenhagen S, editors. Molecular pathogenesis of periodontal disease. Washington: American Society for Microbiology; 1994. p. 247-55.

Hill, Jerome. *Understanding Gum Disease*. West Cornwall, Ct.: Berkshire Press, 1984.

Hillier SL, Martius J, Krohn MJ, Kiviat N, Holmes KK, Eschenbach DA. A case-control study of chorioamnionic infection and histologic chorioamnionitis in prematurity. N Engl J Med 1988 Oct;319(15):972-8.

Hillier SL, Nugent RP, Eschenbach DA, Krohn MA, Gibbs RS, Martin DH, Cotch MF, Edelman R, Pastorek JG 2nd, Rao AV, et al. Association between bacterial vaginosis and preterm delivery of a low-birth-weight infant. The vaginal infections and prematurity study group. N Engl J Med 1995 Dec;333(26):1737-42.

Li Y, Caufield PW. The fidelity of initial acquisition of mutans streptococci by infants from their mothers. J Dent Res 1995 Feb;74(2):681-5.

Löe H, Silness J. Periodontal disease in pregnancy. I. Prevalence and severity. Acta Odontol Scand 1963;21:533-51.

Loesche WJ, Giordona J, Hujoel PP. The utility of the BANA test for monitoring anaerobic infections due to spirochetes *(Treponema denticola)* in periodontal disease. J Dent Res 1990 Oct;69(10):1696-702.

Loesche WJ. The identification of bacteria associated with periodontal disease and dental caries by enzymatic methods. Oral Microbiol Immunol 1986;1:65-70.

National Center for Education in Maternal and Child Health, Inequalities in Access: *Oral Health Services for Children and Adolescents with Special Care Needs,* Georgetown University, October 2000.

National Institute of Dental Research. , 1986–1987. National Institutes of Health, Bethesda, MD 1989.

Offenbacher S, Jared HL, O'Reilly PG, Wells SR, Salvi GE, Lawrence HP, Socransky SS, Beck JD. Potential pathogenic mechanisms of periodontitis associated pregnancy complications. Ann Periodontol 1998 Jul;3(1): 233-50.

Offenbacher S, Katz V, Fertik G, Collins J, Boyd D, Maynor G, McKaig R, Beck J. Periodontal infection as a possible risk factor for preterm low birth weight. J Periodontol 1996 Oct;67(10 Suppl):1103-13.

Offenbacher S, Odle BM, Van Dyke TE. The use of crevicular fluid prostaglandin E2 levels as a predictor of periodontal attachment loss. J Periodontal Res 1986;21:101-12

Page RC, Beck JD. Risk assessment for periodontal diseases. Int Dent J 1997;47:61-87.

Page RC. Periodontal diseases: a new paradigm. J Dent Educ 1998;62:812-21.

Papapanou PN. Risk assessments in the diagnosis and treatment of periodontal diseases. J Dent Educ 1998;62: 822-39.

Saglie FR, Marfany A, Camargo P. Intragingival occurrence of *Actinobacillus actinomycetemcomitans and Bacteroides gingivalis* in active destructive periodontal lesions. J Periodontol 1988 Apr;59(4):259-65.

Salvi GE, Lawrence HP, Offenbacher S, Beck JD. Influence of risk factors on the pathogenesis of periodontitis. Periodontol 2000 1997 Jun;14:173-201.

Scannapieco FA. Position paper of the American Academy of Periodontology: periodontal disease as a potential risk factor for systemic diseases. J Periodontol 1998 Jul;69(7):841-50.

Slots J. Subgingival Microflora and periodontal disease. J.Clin Periodontology 1979;6:351-382

Socransky SS, Haffajee AD. The bacterial etiology of destructive periodontal disease: current concepts. J Periodontol 1992;63:322-31.

Strauss RP, Hunt RJ. Understanding the value of teeth to older adults: influences on the quality of life. J Am Dent Assoc 1993 Jan;124(1):105-10.

Tenovuo J, Häkkinen P, Paunio P, Emilson CG. Effects of chlorhexidine-fluoride gel treatments in mothers on the establishment of mutans streptococci in primary teeth and development of dental caries in children. Caries Res 1992;26:275-80.

U.S. Department of Health and Human Services (USDHHS), Center for Research for Mothers and Children. Public Health Service/National Institutes of Health Progress Report. Washington: U.S. Department of Health and Human Services; 1984.

U.S. Department of Health and Human Services, Health Resources and Services Administration, Maternal Child Health Bureau.

U.S. Department of Health and Human Services. *Oral Health in America: A Report of the Surgeon General.* National Institute of Dental and Craniofacial Research, Rockville, MD, National Institutes of Health, 2000.

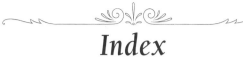

Index

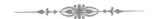

About the Author

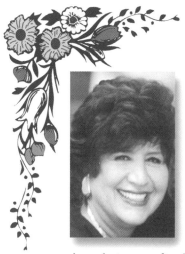

Sheila Wolf, known affectionately by her patients as **Mama Gums**, has been a dental hygienist for 32 years and has helped many hundreds of patients save teeth that were considered "hopeless". Through education, encouragement, and a non-surgical approach to treating gum infections, she has enabled many people to take control of not only their oral health, but their full body health as well. She has taught people the techniques, refined their skills, and advised on the use of many holistic "medications," which empowered them to accomplish what other dental professionals did not think possible.

Sheila has had a passion for helping people since her teens when she had an after-school job as a candy striper (helper) in a local teaching hospital. At 22, she went to Fones School of Dental Hygiene and began teaching oral hygiene to her patients. Since 1973, she has been recognized in her local neighborhoods as a "friend of the Tooth Fairy" who hands out toothbrushes, dental floss, and toothpaste to the children who come to her door on Halloween night. Mothers and fathers are tickled that their goblins are encouraged to clean their teeth after eating their trick-or-treat candies.

In 1982, Sheila volunteered as a "dental nurse" on a Kibbutz in Israel where she began her program of education specifically aimed towards the children, and those adults suffering from advanced gum disease.

In 1991, she met Sister Marie, a teacher from a remote village in Africa, who was on a sabbatical in the United States. Sheila trained her in the "how to" of brushing and flossing to pass on to her children, who had never even seen a brush before. Donations that Sheila obtained from Butler, Crest, and Colgate, outfitted Sister Marie with enough provisions and educational materials to make a real difference to the kids' oral health.

Sheila's most recent adventure was a trip to the Appalachian Mountains to a very underprivileged coal-mining town in Kentucky where she taught oral hygiene in a one-room schoolhouse. Some of the students were so needy that they shared toothbrushes (if they had them at all) with their brothers and sisters. Showing videos of Snoopy's visit to the dentist and Charlie Brown's tooth brushing lesson, demonstrating how to brush and floss, and answering their questions about their mouths, Sheila gave the children an experience they will remember for a long time.

The vision of this book is to reach out to as many people as possible. Sheila has taken time out from her career and has "gone public" to take her message beyond the limited patients whom she could reach in her dental chair. She has brought this information to you so that you may keep your teeth, become healthier, and just possibly add years to your life.

And your baby's...

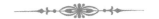

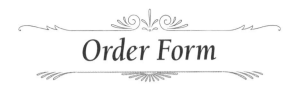

Order Form

Pregnancy and Oral Health
The critical connection between your mouth and your baby

Sheila Wolf, RDH
"Mama Gums"

Please send _____ copies of Pregnancy and Oral Health at $15.95 each.

Name:_____

Address:_____

_____

_____

email:_____ Phone: (_____)_____

How did you hear about this book? _____
Sales tax: Please add $1.05 sales tax for each book on orders shipped to
California addresses.

Shipping (US): $4 for first copy, $2 for each additional book.
Free shipping for orders of 6 or more.

Payment enclosed: $_____

R
Radcliffe Publishing
San Diego, California

PO Box 151708, San Diego, CA 92175-1708, USA.

Share with your friends! Special discounts for large quantities.

For more information visit
www.Mamagums.com or email Mama-Gums@cox.net
or call toll free 866-MamaGums (866-626-2486)

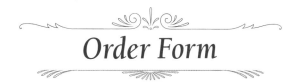

Order Form

Pregnancy and Oral Health
The critical connection between your mouth and your baby

Sheila Wolf, RDH
"Mama Gums"

Please send _____ copies of Pregnancy and Oral Health at $15.95 each.

Name:_____

Address:_____

_____

_____

email:_____ Phone: (_____)_____

How did you hear about this book? _____

Sales tax: Please add $1.05 sales tax for each book on orders shipped to California addresses.

Shipping (US): $4 for first copy, $2 for each additional book.
Free shipping for orders of 6 or more.

Payment enclosed: $_____

R
Radcliffe Publishing
San Diego, California

PO Box 151708, San Diego, CA 92175-1708, USA.

Share with your friends! Special discounts for large quantities.

For more information visit
www.Mamagums.com or email Mama-Gums@cox.net
or call toll free 866-MamaGums (866-626-2486)

*While every effort has been made to make sure
this book is free of errors, realistically, perfection is
unachievable. I invite you to e-mail or write me with
any corrections or suggestions you may have. Your
contribution will be greatly appreciated.*

Thank you.

Mama Gume